Absent Fathers?

Jonathan Bradshaw, Carol Stimson,
Christine Skinner and
Julie Williams

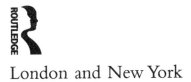

London and New York

First published 1999 by Routledge
11 New Fetter Lane, London EC4P 4EE

Simultaneously published in the USA and Canada
by Routledge
29 West 35th Street, New York, NY 10001

Routledge is an imprint of the Taylor & Francis Group

© 1999 Jonathan Bradshaw, Carol Stimson, Christine Skinner and
Julie Williams

Typeset in Bembo by Graphicraft Limited, Hong Kong
Printed and bound in Great Britain by MPG Books, Bodmin,
Cornwall

British Library Cataloguing in Publication Data
A catalogue record for this book is available from the British Library

Library of Congress Cataloging in Publication Data
Absent fathers? / Jonathan Bradshaw . . . [et al.].
        p.   cm.
    Includes bibliographical references and index.
    ISBN 0-415-21592-7. — ISBN 0-415-21593-5
    1. Absentee fathers—Great Britain Statistics.   2. Custody
of children—Great Britain Statistics.   3. Child support—Great
Britain Statistics.   4. Family life surveys—Great Britain.
I. Bradshaw, Jonathan.
HQ756.8.A25   1999
306.874′2′0941—dc21   99-23942
                                                    CIP

ISBN 0-415-21592-7 (hbk)
ISBN 0-415-21593-5 (pbk)

Absent Fathers?

One of the consequences of the changes that have been taking place in family form in recent decades is that non-resident fathers are now very prevalent. As many as one man in seven between the ages of 16 and 65 is a non-resident father and many others will have experienced living apart from their children. Media and political discourse depict non-resident fathers as feckless 'Deadbeat Dads', but *Absent Fathers?* paints a pervasive picture of men still struggling to be fathers of non-resident children.

Absent Fathers? is based on a national survey of over 600 non-resident fathers in Britain as well as two in-depth studies using qualitative interviews. It explores how men become non-resident fathers and how they feel about it. It then describes their present circumstances and those of their children, and their employment, income and housing circumstances.

More fathers than expected want to have contact and fulfil their parental obligations, social, emotional and financial, but one is unsatisfactory without the others. *Absent Fathers?* suggests that policy makers seeking to enforce financial obligations need to recognise this and the emotional and moral turmoil that follows family separations, cohabitation breakdown or non-marital births.

Jonathan Bradshaw is Professor of Social Policy; **Christine Skinner** is a Research Student; **Julie Williams** is a Research Fellow and they are all at the Social Policy Research Unit, University of York. The late Carol Stimson was a Research Fellow, also at the University of York.

Dedicated to Aidan Stimson (Carol's grandchild)

Contents

13 Concluding discussion   224

     Notes   233
     References and further reading   235
     Index   252

List of figures and tables

Figures

Tables

Preface

All research projects, certainly large empirical projects involving team-work, have a natural history that affects the outcome in some way. In most publications arising from research, this story is never told. The internal discussions about design, method and interpretation, the mistakes, the reasons for delay, tensions between individuals involved and so on – all of these tend to be ignored in the articles, chapters, conference papers and books that are the product of research. There is reason to justify this behind-the-baize-door approach to presenting research. After all, the reader is interested in the findings, not the problems involved in achieving them. To set out to describe the course of the research process in a form other than the limited description of the methods routinely required, is to risk being seen as self-serving and irrelevant.

However, in this project we cannot avoid reporting what a devastating blow was the death of Carol Stimson in a car crash on 9 May 1997. She had been the named research fellow in the application for funding to ESRC. She was then the principal researcher, responsible on a day-to-day basis for the management of the work. She was the one who had done most of the scholarship, much of the thinking, handled the external relations, was most advanced in the writing and was solely responsible for the qualitative part of the study, which focused on relationships between the fathers and their children. She also happened to be the wife of Jonathan Bradshaw, the applicant, responsible for directing the project and for its successful completion.

Carol Stimson had left papers: she had completed the fieldwork and analysis of her qualitative sample; there were drafts of chapters in hard copy and on disk; also a bibliography and parts of a literature review. But those of us who were left to deal with these, as well as being personally devastated by her loss, could not rescue two particular elements of the project and the reader needs to understand this and hopefully make allowances for it.

First, when Carol was drafting the results of her qualitative material we did not yet have all the results of the quantitative part of the project, the sample survey. So she had little opportunity to think about the two together, to review her material and reflect on it in the light of the survey results.

Second, we always knew that combining qualitative and quantitative material in this book was, as ever, going to be very difficult. But we had every intention of attempting it, through a process of discussion, reflection and reconciliation. That required time at the end of the analysis phase of the research, time that was denied to us by her death.

The title of the book

The research project on which this book is based originally had the title *Fathers Apart in Britain*. We preferred it to the tendentious use of 'absent father' in the child support legislation. However, in the course of the project, we became increasingly dissatisfied with 'fathers apart', mainly because it implied a physical and emotional distance between fathers and their children that did not represent what we were finding in the research. We therefore started using 'non-resident fathers' – despite the fact that many of these fathers may be resident for some periods of time with the children who normally live with their mother in another household, as well as, commonly, being a resident social and/or biological father of other children. So although the title of the book is *Absent Fathers?*, we employ the term non-resident fathers throughout the text. It is good to see that in official government documents, for example the Green Paper on Child Support (UK, Cmnd 3992, 1998), 'non-resident' has replaced 'absent'.

Jonathan Bradshaw
Blues Point Road
Sydney
18 February 1998

Acknowledgements

This research was funded by the Economic and Social Research Council as one of the projects (L315 25 3005) in the Programme on Population and Household Change: Demographic Processes and Impacts in the United Kingdom.

Professor Susan McRae was the academic coordinator of the Programme and the liaison staff at ESRC were Margaret Edmonds and Gary Grubb. We are grateful for their support and, in the end, patience, and also to those colleagues who also had projects in the Programme and for the opportunities they gave us to talk about our work.

The Department of Social Security made a generous contribution to the budget in allowing us to expand the sample, and we are grateful to our liaison officers Tony Martin and Dr Dan Murphy.

We are grateful to Siobhan Carey at OPCS and Nick Moon at MORI for managing the fieldwork for the survey.

Sally Pulleyn and Rebecca Harrison improved the manuscript and Janet Moore provided administrative support throughout the project.

We are grateful for the comments we have received from our colleagues at the University of York and especially Dr Dan Meyer, Dr Carol Anne Hooper, Karen Bloor and Anne Corden.

Last, but certainly not least, we are grateful to the many non-resident fathers who took part in this research. We are particularly in their debt for the time they gave to talk to us so freely and about things that were often hard. We are particularly grateful to Richard Oppenheimer and Hugh Burkitt.

1 Introduction

One of the consequences of the changes taking place in family form is the production of non-resident fathers. In the past as today, fathers were more or less temporarily absent from their children as a result of active service in the armed forces, leaving home to find work, undertaking work that took them away from home, imprisonment or hospitalisation. However, today they emerge most commonly in one (or more) of three ways: non-marital births; the breakdown of the relationships of unmarried cohabiting couples with children; or the separation and divorce of married couples with children. Of course all these have been the cause of non-resident fathers in the past, but they are now much more common than they have been.

Non-resident fathers have been depicted in a mainly negative way.[1] In the US, non-resident fathers are frequently called Deadbeat Dads, and in the UK they have been presented as feckless ne'er-do-wells passing on their responsibilities to the taxpayer. Indeed, it was this firm non-resident father ideology that was responsible, to some extent, for the way the Child Support Act 1991 was launched. Margaret Thatcher set the tone of child support policy making in talking about fathers 'walking away from marriage . . . neither maintains nor shows any interest in the child. . . . No father should be able to escape his responsibility . . .' (National Children's Homes George Thomas Society Lecture, 17 January 1990). A few weeks following that lecture, Kenneth Baker, then Chairman of the Conservative Party, reinforced the point – 'Not only is it just that fathers should contribute to the upkeep of their children: it is also crucial that we begin to break the culture which views it as acceptable for a man to walk away from the consequences of his actions in this way. Ensuring that fathers help support the mothers of their children is one way of doing that' (quoted in Burghes, 1991: 6). Peter Lilley in one of his notorious doggerels to the Conservative Party Conference singled out 'Dads who won't support the kids of ladies . . . they have kissed' (7 October 1992).

This negative discourse about non-resident fathers has been part of a wider popular debate about family change, which has vilified both lone mothers and non-resident fathers. In an analysis of ten national daily and ten Sunday newspapers in June 1994, Lloyd (1996) found more items relating to fathers and fatherhood than motherhood or parenting. In the stories, fathers were presented as archetypes – either heroes or monsters (this is similar to Furstenberg's (1988a) delineation of Good Dad/Bad Dad). By far the largest group of monster stories found by Lloyd described them as having either killed, abused or bullied those who were closest to them. He concluded, 'generally fathers are described as problematic. They do not take responsibility for the children they contribute in making, they have little to offer economically (and increasingly in terms of sperm), and they don't contribute to the running of the home or looking after the children and are too often sexually and physically abusive' (p. 4). Song and Edwards (1995) have also investigated the way that black fathers are portrayed in the media. Particularly, following the publication of Augustus' (1995) novel, there has been a good deal of coverage in *Voice*, one of Britain's best black newspapers, about the relationship between 'babymothers' (black women who have children with a number of male partners) and 'babyfathers' (black men who have children with several female partners).

These ideas are reflected not just in the political and media discourse. Academic work has sought to identify them as errant, causal agents for the demise of our social fabric, particularly blaming 'absent fathers' for being inadequate role models for their children, for the poverty of their children and for rising crime rates (Dench, 1994; Dennis and Erdos, 1992; Murray, 1990).

However, the research for this book was motivated by three rather different factors: the very rapid increase in the prevalence of non-resident fathers; the almost complete absence of knowledge about their circumstances; and the fact that they are becoming a focus of policy concerns. Bad policy has already been made (the Child Support Act 1991) and research should contribute to making better policy.

THE PREVALENCE OF NON-RESIDENT FATHERS

The number of fathers who are non-resident has increased very rapidly in the 1980s, and especially the 1990s, and is still increasing. The numbers of non-marital births and relationship breakdowns are still increasing. Haskey (1998) estimates that the number of lone parent families increased to 1.6 million in 1996 from 0.57 million in 1971. These lone parent families contain 2.8 million children. Around 8 per cent of these lone parent families are headed by men. Around 4 per cent of the lone mothers are widows. Some of their unmarried former partners will also have died. The rest all have children with non-resident biological fathers.

However, the prevalence of non-resident fathers is much higher than the number of lone mother families. Most lone mothers repartner and are no longer lone mothers (though they remain parents with care). Haskey (1989a) and Haskey and Kiernan (1989) estimate that two and a half years after divorce a third of women had remarried and another third were cohabiting. But the fathers of lone mothers' children remain non-resident fathers as long as their children are children.

One objective of this research was to produce an estimate of the prevalence of non-resident fathers. For each lone mother there are one or more non-resident fathers. More or less all fathers (and mothers) eventually become non-resident in that their children leave home. We chose an age cut-off in our survey, which is the one used traditionally to define a lone parent (child under 16 or 16–18 inclusive and in full-time education). This is also the one employed in social policy – child benefit is payable on that basis. Also under the Child Support Act 1991 parents are no longer required to pay child support when the youngest child is no longer under the age of 19 (i.e. including their eighteenth year). But it is arguable that in the context of older and later transitions from the parental home, 18 is far too early a cut-off. Certainly there are dependent children living with their (lone) mothers long after the age of 18, and they have non-resident fathers – who have not been covered in this study.

Another reason for not basing estimates of the prevalence of non-resident fathers on the prevalence of lone mothers is the fact that Bradshaw and Millar (1991) found that their sample of lone mothers contained a proportion of children derived from more than one partnership. In fact about 7 per cent of lone parents had had at least one child by a second child-bearing relationship; 1 per cent had a child from a third child-bearing relationship; and five lone parents had had at least one child from a fourth child-bearing relationship (no one in the sample had had more than four child-bearing relationships). Similarly, as we shall see, 11 per cent of fathers in this study admitted to having had children with more than one partner and 3 per cent had fathered children with three or more partners.

Then there is the really difficult problem in making an estimate of prevalence. There are undoubtably fathers who do not know they are the father of a child, fathers who think they are the father of a child but are not, and mothers who think wrongly that a certain man is the father of their child when he is not. Some insights into this are found in the experience of the Child Support Agency. At November 1995 there were 11,464 disputed paternity cases pending and a further 904 cases where tests had been completed (Hansard, 2 February 1996, cols. 991 and 993). This represents 2.5 per cent of all the 'live' cases of the agency at that time. The Network Against the Child Support Act (NACSA) (later to rename itself the National Association for Child Support Action) has estimated that some 14 per cent of the completed DNA tests have proved that the man is not the father of the child(ren) (*NACSA News*, March 1996); it is not clear, however, on what basis NACSA arrived at this estimate. Coleman (1996) reports that a review of false paternity data for the US gives a range of 2.1 to 11.8 per cent, but figures based on cystic fibrosis cases found only 1.4 per cent of false paternity cases for the UK. Clarke (1997) suggests from her analysis of the British Household Panel Survey (BHPS) that under-reporting of male fertility runs between 10 and 15 per cent of births and up to 30 to 50 per cent of non-marital births.

Given these problems, it is difficult to produce reasonable estimates of the number of non-resident fathers in Britain. Certainly there are over two million and there could be as many as five million. Perhaps the best way to think about the scale of the experience of non-resident fathering is to note the fact that it is estimated that between a third and half of all children will experience a period of not living with both natural parents during their childhood. Each one of those children will have a non-resident parent and in most cases it will be the father.

Previous research

Despite their prevalence, despite the plethora of research that is now available on lone parent families (for a recent review see Ford and Millar, 1998), despite the hugely expanding literature on fathering and fatherhood (for recent reviews see Burghes, Clarke and Cronin, 1997; Popay, Hearn and Edwards, 1998), up to now very little is known about the circumstances of non-resident fathers. Unlike lone mothers, as a group they are not particularly likely to be dependent on public services (at least as non-resident fathers). Partly for that reason they are difficult to identify. There is no register of them – birth registration records provide details of fathers only for births to married couples and jointly registered births outside marriage. Therefore very little basic information about the fertility history of men has ever been collected, and there is practically no basic demographic information about non-resident fathers.

There have been two large-scale longitudinal studies in the United States that tried to obtain representative samples of non-resident fathers[2], and recently published is a major new study (Garfinkel *et al.*, 1998). The issue of non-resident fathers in the United States is just as salient as it is in the UK. But the characteristics of non-resident fathers (and lone parents) in the US are very different to those in the UK and so is the context in which policy is made. So we cannot rely on US data for policy making in the UK.

In the UK there has been no previous attempt to study a representative sample of non-resident fathers. That does not mean that nothing is known about them. Studies of lone parents have asked questions of the lone mothers about the fathers of their children (Bradshaw and Millar, 1991; Ford, Marsh and Finlayson, 1998; Ford, Marsh and McKay, 1995; McKay and Marsh, 1994; Marsh and McKay, 1993) and some of this information will be referred to later. Burgoyne and Millar (1994) undertook a follow-up study of a small sample of fathers identified in the Bradshaw and Millar (1991) lone parents survey. When the Department of Social Security (DSS) came to design the Child Support Act they discovered that practically nothing was known about 'absent fathers'. The White Paper (UK, Cmnd 1264, 1990) drew extensively on drafts of Bradshaw and Millar (1991) and also undertook a sample survey of maintenance cases settled in the courts.

Prior to the start of the research reported here, there had been only one other British source of information on non-resident fathers. At the request of the DSS, Marsh (1993) undertook some secondary analysis of non-resident parents in the 1991 survey of the National Child Development Survey (NCDS) when the 1958 birth cohort were 33 years old.[3] He found that nearly 6 per cent of parents and 8 per cent of men admitted to having a child living in another household. The survey covered only 70 per cent of the original sample of 16,500 children and Marsh took the view that about a third of non-resident fathers were missed by the survey, partly due to bias in attrition.

Since this project began, some useful additional sources of information on non-resident fathers have been produced. Simpson, McCarthy and Walker (1995) have published their study of the experiences of ninety-one fathers who were in the process of divorce, having followed them for five years. Maclean and Eekelaar (1997) published their investigation into the views of 250 parents, identified by using methods similar to those used in this study. But only fifty-five of their sample were non-resident parents and only forty-nine of them were men. Burghes,

Clarke and Cronin (1997) undertook an analysis of the BHPS 1992 and found that 15.2 per cent of all fathers aged 16–64 had children under 18 living in another household. Because 35.2 per cent of men aged 16–64 are fathers, they estimate that 5.4 per cent of men aged 16–64 have at least one child under 18 in another household (4.6 to 6.1 are the 95 per cent confidence limits). Finally, McKay, using the Family and Working Lives Survey (FWLS) to trace family change, found 268 cases, 5.6 per cent of the men aged 16–69, who had non-resident children.[4] (Also 2.8 per cent of women could be described as non-resident mothers.) McKay undertook some analysis of the characteristics of these fathers and these are used to compare with our sample in the next chapter.

Policy concerns

Non-resident fathers have increasingly become the focus of policy concerns in the 1980s and 1990s, particularly in relation to family law and child support. Social policy has been slow to come to terms with and respond to the changes that have taken place in family form in the past three decades. Policy has been motivated by a variety of sometimes conflicting concerns. In relation to non-resident fathers they have included:

- the high proportion of lone mothers dependent on Income Support and other benefits and the increasing cost;
- evidence of the bleak state of the living standards of lone mothers and their children, and that after relationship breakdown, on average, lone mothers end up poorer than non-resident fathers;
- evidence that many fathers are not providing any financial support for their children (and former partners) and others are only providing small amounts, often episodically;
- evidence that fathers are losing contact with their children after relationship breakdown and anxiety that this is not in the best interest of the child, the father or the taxpayer;
- knowledge that no arrangements are in place for recognising the father of a child born outside marriage (paternity can only be recognised if the child is jointly registered in the names of the father and the mother, and this can only be done with the mother's agreement). Unmarried fathers still do not have the same rights as married fathers, and neither do their children; and
- the law governing the dissolution of married partnerships does not cover the dissolution of cohabiting partnerships; and anyway it is not geared to produce agreed outcomes covering property, child support, contact, pensions and other matters.

Some of these issues have been tackled in legislation in recent years, including the Family Law Reform Act 1987, the Children Act 1989, the Human Fertilisation and Embryology Act 1990, the Family Law Act 1997, the 1991 and 1995 Child Support Acts, and further legislation is planned covering pension rights on divorce, child support and the rights of unmarried fathers.

However, there remains a good deal of confusion about what should be appropriate policy responses to the increase in non-resident fathers. These are familiar dilemmas in social policy – about the appropriate balance between private and public responsibilities, whether and how public policy should seek to structure or influence private behaviour, and the balance between the rights and responsibilities of parents, children and the public. However, clear thought and sensible policy have been hampered by a lack of knowledge.

This study

The objectives of this study are to contribute to knowledge about the circumstances of non-resident fathers in Britain. We also hope to contribute to the understanding of the nature of fathering in modern Britain and to inform policy making on maintenance, conciliation and social security and thereby produce a companion baseline survey to that provided by *Lone Parent Families in the UK* (Bradshaw and Millar, 1991).

The material collected was obtained using a sample survey of non-resident fathers in Britain, and in-depth interviews with fathers in two subsamples from the main survey, one focusing on the issue of contact and the other on financial support. Chapter 2 describes the methods employed in these studies in more detail. Chapter 3 uses the data from the survey to explore the backgrounds of the men and the processes that led them to become non-resident fathers and examines their present family and household circumstances, drawing on both the survey and some of the qualitative material. The next two chapters are based on the survey and cover the non-resident fathers' employment and income (Chapter 4), and housing (Chapter 5). The next two chapters concentrate on the contact that the fathers have with their children using the quantitative material (Chapter 6) and the qualitative material (Chapter 7). The next five chapters focus on financial support: Chapter 8 uses the survey to establish who pays child support and Chapter 9 analyses the level of child support paid, and the level of informal support. Chapter 10 uses both the survey and the qualitative study to examine the fathers' experiences of the Child Support Agency. Chapters 11 and 12 draw entirely on the qualitative data to examine, in depth, the fathers' feelings about their financial obligations and what determines them. Chapter 13 concludes the study. In the tables in which our findings are summarised, figures for percentages are rounded off to whole numbers, with the occasional result that the total may appear to be slightly above or below 100 per cent.

2 Methods of collecting the data

INTRODUCTION

It was always envisaged that fathers living apart from their children would be a particularly difficult population to study. This expectation has been proved correct. In this chapter we describe how the sample for the survey was identified, compare the characteristics of those who were eventually interviewed with those who identified themselves as having children in another household, but were not interviewed, and draw some conclusions about the bias in the resultant sample of fathers, and make corrections for this. We compare the characteristics of our sample with the characteristics of other samples of non-resident fathers. Finally we present the design of the two qualitative studies undertaken of subsamples from the main survey.

THE SAMPLE SURVEY

This study sought to interview a representative sample of fathers living apart from their children. There was no satisfactory sampling frame for such a sample. Because non-resident fathers are not as a group dependent on public services, it was not possible to use public records (for example, benefit data) as a sampling frame, as have been used to investigate lone parent families (for example Bradshaw and Millar, 1991). One possibility was to mount a screening survey. But a purpose-built screening survey would have been very large and very costly. Instead it was decided to use omnibus surveys as a vehicle for identifying non-resident fathers. There were three survey companies at the time the study was designed which operated omnibus surveys of representative samples of individuals – National Opinion Polls (NOP), the Office of Population Censuses and Surveys (OPCS) and Research Services of

Great Britain (RSGB). Tenders were sought from all three companies. RSGB came through with a quotation that was substantially higher than the other firms and out of reach of the budget. It was therefore decided to go ahead with the two other companies. This was unfortunate, as RSGB had by far the largest omnibus, and if they had been involved in the study it would have been possible to pick up the sample rather more quickly than it turned out. NOP kindly tried out a screening question as a pilot exercise in their omnibus survey in January 1995. They found that 4 per cent of men identified themselves as nonresident fathers and about 60 per cent of those said that they would be prepared to be interviewed. On this basis it was estimated that it would be possible to achieve a sample of 1,000 non-resident fathers by employing the OPCS and NOP omnibus for a period of ten months.

Screening began in April 1995. Each man between the ages of 16 and 65 was asked the following question:

> Are you the father of a child under 16, or between 16 and 18 and in full time education, who normally lives with their mother in another household?

If they answered yes, they were asked if they would be willing to be interviewed.

The screening question appeared to be understood (though in the end, completed questionnaires were received for twenty-nine men who no longer had a dependent child living in another household). It can be seen from Table 2.1 that NOP, whose omnibus was three times the size of OPCS, screened 25,824 men and OPCS screened 8,134 men. Both agencies achieved a similar proportion of men identifying themselves as the father of a child living with their mother in another household. However, OPCS obtained agreement to an interview from 56 per cent of non-resident fathers identified, and achieved interviews with all of them. In contrast, NOP obtained agreement with only 40 per cent of the fathers identified, and only achieved interviews with 30 per cent. It appears that there are two reasons for this substantial difference between the achievements of the companies. OPCS interviewers used paper and pencil for both their omnibus survey and the follow-up survey and they also used the same interviewers. Thus they were able to obtain the interview with fathers who assented to be interviewed, for the most part, immediately after they were identified in the omnibus screen. NOP, in contrast, used computer aided interviewing (CAPI) for both their omnibus and their follow-up interview. The omnibus field force were only able to identify the non-resident fathers, and a separate interview, with a different laptop computer, often using a different interviewer, had to be arranged for the follow-up. Often there were considerable delays between identifying non-resident fathers, and interviewing them. The result was a very poor rate of interviews achieved by NOP. This resulted in an overall response rate of 84 per cent of the non-resident fathers who agreed to be interviewed but only 38 per cent of those identified by the screen.

Table 2.1 Response to the screening survey and follow-up survey

	NOP	OPCS	Total
Number of men screened	25,824	8,134	33,958
Non-resident fathers identified	1,186	464	1,650
(% of the men screened)	(4.6%)	(5.7%)	(4.9%)
Non-resident fathers agreeing to an interview	477	258	735
(% of those identified)	(40%)	(56%)	(45%)
Interviews achieved (% of non-resident fathers identified)	361	258	619
	(30%)	(56%)	(38%)

Unfortunately NOP had by far the largest screen, and their failure to achieve interviews with all the fathers identified resulted in the sample size building up much more slowly than expected. The screening period was extended until the end of 1995, and then until the end of April 1996. This meant that the follow-up interviews were not completed by NOP until August 1996, and a clean data tape was not received until November 1996 – more than six months later than envisaged. The sample was still short of the target of 1,000 non-resident fathers.

So the achieved sample is smaller than was intended, and the response rate, at least by NOP, was lower than expected. Nevertheless the question remains: Is the achieved sample representative?

Testing the representativeness of the sample

In this survey there are six possible sources of unrepresentativeness:

1   Sampling error. No sample fully represents the population from which it is drawn. This is as true for this sample as any other, and thankfully sampling theory makes it possible to predict the likely sampling error in a sample. Sampling error in this study will have occurred at the omnibus survey and at the follow-up stage.

2   However, there is likely to be an under-representation of non-resident fathers in the omnibus surveys. This observation is derived from the work of Rendall *et al.* (1997) on the incomplete reporting of male fertility in the British Household Panel Survey (BHPS) and

the US Panel Study of Income Dynamics. For example, using data on male and female fertility collected in 1992 in the BHPS, they found that 11.5 per cent of male fertility was missing and 60 per cent of this was due to under-representation in the sample rather than non-reporting. They also found a much higher proportion of missing male fertility among non-marital births and marital births where the marriage was no longer intact at the survey date (approximately 19 per cent of the total in the BHPS). Among the non-marital births, 36 per cent of male fertility was missing though less than a quarter (23 per cent) of it could be attributed to under-representation in the sample – the rest was due to non-reporting. However, 40 per cent of non-intact marital births were missing and 64 per cent of these were due to under-representation in the sample. This suggests that non-resident fathers are likely to be under-represented in the omnibus surveys.

3   Some of the men who were asked whether they were the father of a child living in another household replied 'no' wrongly, because they did not know that they were. There is no way that this source of bias can be dealt with.

4   Some of the men who were asked whether they were the father of a child living in another household answered 'no' wrongly, because they did not want to admit it or acknowledge it. In the context of the public controversy over the Child Support Agency, the bad press that non-resident fathers were getting (discussed in Chapter 1) and a general anxiety about their self-image, it is inevitable that there would be fathers in this category. Given how little is known about the prevalence of non-resident fathers, it is difficult to be certain how big this group is. Of the men screened, 4.9 per cent said that they were non-resident fathers. This is considerably lower than the 8 per cent of men identified by Marsh (1993) using the National Child Development Study, but it is similar (within the 95 per cent confidence limits) to the 5.4 per cent found by Burghes, Clarke and Cronin (1997) in the British Household Panel Survey, and similar to the 5.6 per cent found by McKay (personal communication) in the survey of Family and Working Lives. However, 5 per cent of men aged 16–65 represents only around one million men out of around 18 million men in Britain in that age range. If we are correct in our conclusion that there are more than two million non-resident fathers, and there may be as many as five million, then we are a long way short of identifying all the non-resident fathers in the population for this study. This fact needs to be borne in mind in considering the findings in the rest of the book.

There is no way that this source of bias can be dealt with. It is only possible to speculate about the characteristics of those men who did not know or who failed to admit that they were the fathers of children whom they were not living with. One can suggest that they were probably more likely to have been the fathers of children born outside marriage and cohabitation, where the relationship with the mother was fleeting or at least where they were not living together. It is also possible that they would probably be men who were likely to have to be interviewed in the presence of new wives/partners/relations and therefore did not feel able to be as frank as they might otherwise have been. As we have seen from the work of Rendall *et al.* (1997) in the BHPS it is estimated that there is a deficit of 36 per cent of non-marital births and 77 per cent of these are due to non-reporting by fathers, whereas there is a deficit of 40 per cent of non-intact marital births and 36 per cent of them are due to non-reporting. This suggests that single non-resident fathers are less likely to report that they are fathers.

5 Some of the men who acknowledged that they were the father of a child living in another household refused a follow-up interview. To some extent the possible effects of this source of bias can be described because the agencies provided data on all respondents to their omnibus survey, whether or not they were interviewed as part of the follow-up survey.

6 Some of the men who acknowledged that they were the father of a child living in another household and who agreed to be interviewed were never interviewed. This is a problem for the NOP sample and again the possible effects of this source of bias can be described using the omnibus survey.

A great deal more can be discovered about the characteristics of those men who identified themselves as non-resident fathers but for whom a follow-up interview was not obtained because they either refused (group 5 above) or the survey agency failed to achieve one (group 6 above). The next section explores this source of bias.

Comparing respondents and non-respondents

All omnibus surveys collect standard data on the characteristics of their samples. The standard data collected by NOP and OPCS are not identical, but with a modest amount of manipulation it was possible to combine the two data sets for most relevant variables.[5]

Table 2.2 Results of a logistic regression of the odds of being interviewed

Variable	N	Bivariate	N	Simultaneous	Best Fitting
	1650		1562		
Marital status					
married	467	1.00	447	1.00	1.00
living as married	244	1.58★★	236	1.54★	1.58★★
single	269	0.64★★	249	0.82	0.77
separated	210	1.11	203	1.24	1.25
divorced	454	1.52★★	427	1.62★	1.67★★★
Age left full-time education					
under 15	476	1.00	454	1.00	
16	736	1.11	696	1.11	
over 16	436	1.44★★	412	1.20	
Cars					
none	515	1.00	481	1.00	
one	820	1.27★	783	1.07	
two or more	310	1.58★★	298	1.50★	
Age					
16–30	334	1.00	311	1.00	
31–34	297	1.62★★	284	1.23	
35–40	439	1.67★★★	412	1.21	
41+	577	1.60★★	555	1.18	
Employment status					
employed	894	1.00	857	1.00	
self-employed	199	1.00	191	0.89	
inactive	550	0.74★★	514	0.82	
Economic status					
working	1,098	1.00	1,051	1.00	
unemployed	329	0.65★★	308	1.36	
inactive	217	0.89	203	1.51	
Class					
professional/intermediate	254	1.00	247	1.00	1.00
skilled non-manual	267	0.72	257	0.81	0.77
skilled manual	468	0.76	448	0.95	0.83
partly skilled	315	0.66★	299	0.86	0.72
unskilled	329	0.44★★★	311	0.53★★	0.48★★★
Tenure					
owns outright	146	1.00	145	1.00	
owns with mortgage	712	1.17	698	0.96	
rents LA/HA	465	0.92	450	0.98	
private rent	271	0.92	269	0.86	
Number in household					
1	588	1.00	557	1.00	
2	405	1.05	382	1.02	
3	285	0.85	270	0.85	
4	226	0.83	216	0.82	
5 or more	146	0.67★	137	0.79	

Table 2.2 (cont'd)

Variable	N	Bivariate	N	Simultaneous	Best Fitting
	1650		1562		
Children					
yes	511	0.87	485	1.04	
no	1,139	1.00	1,077	1.00	
Head of household male					
yes	1,400	1.00	1,332	1.00	
no	248	0.69★	230	0.71	

★p < 0.05; ★★p < 0.01; ★★★p < 0.001; ns p > 0.05

There was no significant difference between the interviewed and the not-interviewed in respect of the gender of the household head, tenure, number of people in the household, children in the household, and gross income.

However, the sample who agreed to be interviewed were statistically less likely than those who were not, to be single, unskilled manual, an employee and under 30.

These characteristics are likely to interact, and therefore a logistic regression was undertaken of the odds of being interviewed to establish the nature of these interactions. The results are summarised in Table 2.2. In the best-fitting model, after controlling for other characteristics, the sample who were interviewed were only significantly different from those who were not interviewed in respect of marital status and social class.[6] The data were therefore weighted by these variables, using as weights the proportion in each marital status/social class cell,[7] for the whole sample identified as non-resident fathers.[8] This weighting procedure resulted in adjusting the characteristics of the interviewees so that there were no longer any significant differences between them and the total identified as non-resident fathers.

Weighting in this way compensates for known response bias, but it does not account for unknown response bias, nor for any bias in the sample of men who identified themselves as non-resident fathers, and this needs to be borne in mind in considering the results in the rest of this book.

In order to check whether any of the response bias was a function of the differences in the success of the survey agencies in achieving interviews with the men whom they had identified as non-resident fathers, we compared the characteristics of the respondents produced by each agency. On most variables, the two samples are surprisingly similar (given the size of the samples and the inevitable sampling error).

Comparisons between our sample and other samples

There are only two sources against which it is possible to check the characteristics of the achieved sample. The first is the special analysis of the Family and Working Lives Survey (FWLS) undertaken by McKay. However, it is important to remember that that survey will also suffer from men not knowing or being willing to acknowledge that they are non-resident fathers, as well as from response bias. Also the subsample of men who identified themselves as non-resident fathers is smaller than in this study – only 268. Nevertheless the characteristics of the non-resident fathers in the samples were remarkably similar. Only two differences are larger than you would expect to obtain due to sampling error. First, current marital status – there were more single men and fewer married men in our sample than in the FWLS sample. This may be due to differences in definitions between the surveys – single in our survey is defined as having no partner in the household, whereas married are married *and* have a partner in the household. Second, the age of the youngest absent child – fewer 11–18 year olds in our sample. This is explainable by the difference in the age cut-off in the FWLS survey, which includes all children up to age 18, whereas we included children over 16 if they were in full-time education.

The second source of comparative data is the Client Satisfaction Survey, undertaken on behalf of the Child Support Agency. Of course its major flaw is that it is a survey of clients who may not necessarily be representative of all non-resident fathers. Nevertheless it is a large sample, and the published report presents a profile of some demographic, housing and educational characteristics of the non-resident parents (96 per cent of whom are fathers) for which we have comparable data. Again the characteristics of the CSA sample are, in most respects, remarkably similar to our sample of non-resident fathers.

METHODS EMPLOYED IN THE QUALITATIVE STUDIES

The research design also included two in-depth qualitative studies, using two different samples. One focused primarily on fathers' active relationships with children and their experiences of contact, and twenty fathers made up this sample. The other focused on fathers' financial obligations among a separate sample of eighteen fathers. The quantitative study was designed to investigate large-scale structural features of the lives of fathers living apart from their children, whereas the qualitative studies were designed to identify the context in which the fathers operate, and to provide a greater understanding of how family life was both perceived and experienced by individual non-resident fathers. Combining different research strategies is not without its inherent problems, as has been commented on by various researchers (Brannen, 1992; Bryman, 1992). Bryman (1992) discusses the different ways of combining research methods and the different weight that is given to each contribution. He suggests that quantitative approaches allow researchers to establish relationships between variables, but they are often weak when it comes to explaining the how and why of these relationships. Qualitative methods on the other hand can be used to explain those relationships.

Ideally the respondents for the in-depth studies should have been chosen following completion of the analysis of the quantitative data, which would have clearly identified relationships among key variables for deeper exploration. However, to avoid losing respondents, it was decided to embark upon the qualitative interviews as soon as possible following the survey interviews. Despite this loss of advantage from the quantitative data analysis, both studies were informed by literature reviews and a small qualitative pilot study with seven non-resident fathers conducted in 1994 (Skinner, 1994). These had identified key areas of concerns for fathers in their relationships with children and their financial obligations.

Choosing respondents for the qualitative studies

Respondents for both the qualitative studies were chosen from those fathers who had taken part in the national survey, and who had agreed to a second interview. The final samples of respondents therefore came from a wide geographical spread from Edinburgh in the north to Brighton in the south. Respondents were contacted by letter directly by the researchers, and written consent for a re-interview was sought. Thereafter interviews were arranged by telephone. However, because the focuses of enquiry of the two studies were distinct, different selection criteria were used for each; these will be discussed in turn.

Qualitative study on father's active relationships with children

Selection criteria and rationale

Previous research on non-resident fathers has concentrated on the immediate post-separation/divorce period. This has been documented by Wallerstein and Blakeslee (1989) and others, as being a difficult time for the family. It is a time when both partners are likely to be suffering from emotional disturbance to some degree, and are not functioning well as parents. We wanted to avoid this traumatic stage in the reaction to the breakup of the family, and to interview fathers when life was beginning to settle into a pattern, to see how they had reorganised and reconstructed their lives, particularly in relation to contact with their children. The sampling frame for this study was constructed by following up only fathers who had been separated for two years or more and who had remained in contact with their children.

Sample size

Names and addresses of fathers who fulfilled these criteria were sought from the market research agencies while they were still conducting the survey. In total, seventy-six fathers fulfilled the selection criteria. The final sample where interviews were achieved comprised the first fathers who agreed to a further interview – a total number of twenty, thirteen from NOP and seven from OPCS.

Qualitative study on fathers' financial obligations

Selection criteria

The advantage of choosing respondents from the national survey for the second qualitative study meant it was possible to be 'judicious' in the selection of cases to allow comparisons to be made between sharply differentiated groups (Bryman, 1992). However, given the need to re-interview respondents as soon as possible, without the benefit of information from the data analysis, the selection criteria used were necessarily cruder than might have been desired. Nonetheless they were good enough to capture a wide diversity in individual circumstances, which could still be contrasted and compared. Unlike the qualitative study on contact, the sampling frame used for financial obligations related to respondents' contacted by only one agency – NOP. A purposive sample was selected from NOP on the basis of respondents' consent to be contacted again, that they had not been selected for the other qualitative study, and on two other dimensions – contact with children and maintenance payments.

This produced four distinctive groups of fathers on the basis of their contact and maintenance, shown in Table 2.3.

Table 2.3 Groups of fathers

Group One	Fathers with regular contact★ and currently paying maintenance.
Group Two	Fathers with regular contact★ but not currently paying maintenance.
Group Three	Fathers with no contact★★ and currently paying maintenance.
Group Four	Fathers with no contact★★ and not currently paying maintenance.

★ Regular contact was defined as ranging from at least once every three months up to daily contact.
★★ No contact was defined as a father having not seen his child at all in the preceding 12 months.

Rationale for constructing a purposive sample

The rationale for choosing fathers for the study on financial obligations was that these two dimensions – contact and maintenance – could act as indicators of fathers' social and financial involvement in their children's lives and hence perhaps also be indicators of fathers' levels of commitment to children. Accordingly fathers in Group One who were in regular contact and paying maintenance might represent fathers who are most involved and committed to their children. Fathers in Group Four who had no contact and were not paying maintenance might represent the opposite extreme. In the two middle groups, where there was a mix of financial and social support, fathers' levels of involvement and commitment to children are more ambiguous. For example, fathers who pay maintenance but have no contact may only be doing so because they are legally forced to pay maintenance. Thus their level of commitment may be very minimal even though they financially provide. Equally, fathers in regular contact but not currently paying maintenance may be willing to provide maintenance, but are either 'unable' to pay or feel they cannot 'afford' to do so. Thus their level of commitment may be very substantial even though they do not pay formal maintenance. It became apparent that when the final sample was achieved and interviews undertaken, the maintenance and contact status of some of the fathers had changed since the time of the original survey questionnaire. This did not present any difficulties, as the group as a whole remained differentiated enough to make comparisons in analysis, but the analysis did not contrast the experiences of the respondents on the basis of the four groups described above (see Chapter 13 for discussion of analysis process).

Sample size

Sixty-eight names and addresses of fathers for the quota sample were received in April 1996. Of those, forty-nine were highlighted as being most viable due to ease of access and having full and correct details. Only forty were actually contacted by letter. Some twelve fathers agreed to be interviewed after the initial contact by letter and a further eight agreed to be interviewed after making contact a second time, either by phone or by letter or a mixture of both. In total, nineteen interviews were conducted among the twenty fathers who agreed to be interviewed. However, one interview was not viable due to technical difficulties, leaving eighteen interviews for analysis. The most difficult groups to achieve interviews with were those fathers who were not paying maintenance (Groups Two and Four), although Group Two was the worst. The reasons for this were not clear, but it could be that these fathers were unwilling to participate because of the stigmatisation surrounding non-payment of maintenance.

Interviews

Both qualitative studies used a semi-structured interview technique utilising a topic guide. The definition of a semi-structured interview was:

> organised around issues of particular interest, while still allowing considerable flexibility in scope and depth.
>
> (May, 1991: 191)

This allowed for consistency in depth but was flexible enough for individual respondents to highlight issues most salient to them.

There was considerable overlap between the studies in terms of the topics covered. For example, the study exploring fathers' relationships with children considered some financial aspects such as the breadwinner role of fathers, while the study on financial obligations also considered issues surrounding contact with children. But they differed in terms of their main focus and emphasis. In the study on fathers' relationships with children three main time-scales were covered: early family life; life in the partnership with the child's mother; and life in the present. The fathers were asked to retrospectively recall their early memories of their original families and their relationships with their father and how much this had influenced their own fathering either positively or negatively. They were also asked to talk about daily living, both in the present and in the past during the cohabitation/marriage. The importance of the breadwinner role was examined, concentrating on its relevance to non-resident fathering. But the focus of the study was the father's contact and relationship with his children, and how far this relationship was influenced by the father's relationship with his ex-partner. In contrast, the study on financial obligations focused more on recent events that directly related to the history of past partnership(s) rather than exploring fatherhood or kin relationships more generally, or over the lifetime of the respondents.

Sensitive topics

Both studies were dealing with highly sensitive topics and this did cause distress for some fathers during the interviews. There was an added dimension of sensitivity for the study on financial obligations – where discussing income/money has perhaps become more of a taboo in modern society than discussing people's sexual relationships. Moreover, money in the form of maintenance (or its lack) has been used in political discourses to stigmatise and criticise the whole population of non-resident fathers.

Data collection and analysis

Data collection was by means of audio tape recording and pen and paper for note taking – notes were taken of factual circumstances such as numbers and ages of children and marital status and current house-hold circumstances, and so on. When the interview formally finished (when the recorder was switched off) field notes were recorded retro-spectively noting the content of the conversation up to the time of departure. General fieldwork notes were also kept, which recorded the interviewers' and the respondents' emotional status prior to, during and following the interview. Also recorded were the interviewers' percep-tions of how 'engaged' both the respondent and the interviewer had been during the interview itself.

Initially tapes were transcribed as soon as possible following the inter-view and themes and categories were identified as part of the transcrip-tion process. Although these emergent themes and categories were not systematically tested in subsequent interviews, they did not change the direction of the studies as suggested by the Grounded Theory method (Bryman, 1992: 84). What the identification of themes achieved was to 'sensitise' the interviewer to the nature of some of the topics raised by fathers.

SUMMARY

There is no doubt that it is particularly hard to obtain a representative sample of non-resident fathers. The problem was not eased by NOP, which obtained a low agreement rate and a poor interview rate, even among those fathers who agreed to be interviewed. Clearly experience now teaches us that, if an omnibus survey is to be used to identify subsamples of the population, it is undesirable to separate the screening interview from the follow-up interview. Given the response rate of only 38 per cent of those men who identified themselves as non-resident fathers, we have been at pains in this chapter to explore response bias first, by comparing the characteristics of respondents and non-respondents. From this it was concluded that the sample was biased in respect of marital status and social class – lacking enough single, unskilled working-class and unemployed men. We were able to adjust for this bias by reweighting. The resulting sample was at least representative of those who in the omnibus screen had identified themselves as non-resident fathers – though not necessarily representative of those who did not know they were non-resident fathers or who did not want to identify themselves. Second, we then compared the sample with two other available sources of information on the characteristics of non-resident fathers and were reassured to find that our sample was remarkably similar (and where it was not, there were reasonable explanations).

However, there is still reason to be cautious about the representativeness of the sample in this study. As we have seen, there has been a mood of vilification of non-resident fathers in Britain in recent years. This has coincided with the Child Support Agency seeking to identify men liable to pay child support. As we shall see, there is also a great sadness and sense of loss among these men. All these may be reasons to expect many men not to identify themselves in the screening survey. It is difficult to establish the prevalence of non-resident fathers, but it is probable that less than half of the non-resident fathers in the omnibus survey acknowledged the fact. This has to be borne in mind in considering the quantitative findings in the rest of this book. Nevertheless, the qualitative studies enrich the survey results and provide insights into processes, experiences, values and attitudes in relation to what it means to be a non-resident father.

3 The characteristics of non-resident fathers

INTRODUCTION

In this chapter we begin the analysis of the results of the survey by exploring how men become non-resident fathers. We also draw on some of the interview material from the qualitative study of contact, which provides a more detailed picture. Then we describe the characteristics of non-resident fathers at the time of their interview.

BECOMING A NON-RESIDENT FATHER

As we have already said, there are only three routes to becoming a non-resident father: a single man can have a sexual encounter with a woman that results in her becoming pregnant and carrying the baby to term; a married couple may separate after a child or children have been born to the marriage, or after the wife is pregnant; and a cohabiting couple may separate from each other, either after the birth of a child or after the female partner is pregnant. In this sample 10 per cent of non-resident fathers had been single, 67 per cent had been married and 23 per cent had been cohabiting.

However, family life is not as simple as this, and the actual experiences of the non-resident fathers are a good deal more complex than this. For a start, the classification of marital status at birth, outlined above, is based on the most recent or only relationship that involved children who were not living with the fathers. In fact sixty-one (10 per cent) of the fathers in this study had had more than one such relationship – fifty-four had had two, four had had three and three had had four. Furthermore their fertility history was not yet over, in the sense that many were now, or would be, in new relationships that might involve the birth of children and these might founder. So the sample is really a truncated portion of the full lives of non-resident fathers. If account is taken of these different relationships involving children, then the proportion in which the father was single is 11 per cent, cohabiting 23 per cent and married 66 per cent. The most common pattern of multiple relationships involving the birth of a child, who was now absent from the father's household, was a married relationship followed by a cohabitation. The next most common was a marriage followed by another marriage.

Table 3.1 shows the relationship status (not formal marital status) of the non-resident fathers at the birth of their first or only absent child, and at the time of the interview. At the time of the interview the largest group were those who were divorced from a previous marriage (25 per cent). Most men were now single (58 per cent), 24 per cent were married and 18 per cent were cohabiting. However, again this hides the real complexity of the status of the fathers. The large group of singles includes the previously single, the ex-married (some of whom are now separated and some divorced) and the ex-cohabiting. Also, between these points in time many of these men may have passed through other relationships, a few of which involved the birth of a child who was now absent from the father's home.

Table 3.1 Relationship status at the time of the interview compared with relationship status to the mother of the youngest non-resident child

Relationship status to the mother of the youngest non-resident child	Percentage of the total %	Relationship status now	Percentage of the total %
Single	9.8	Single	7.5
		Married	1.0
		Cohabiting	1.3
Married	66.9	Single and separated	9.5
		Single and divorced	24.9
		Remarried	19.0
		Cohabiting	13.5
Cohabiting	23.3	Single	16.1
		Married	4.2
		Cohabiting	3.0
Total N = 590	100.0		100.0

Length of time as a non-resident father

Because of these complexities it is somewhat difficult to calculate the length of time that fathers had been living apart from their children.

Table 3.2 Time since separation, by marital status

	Ex-married %	Ex-cohabiting %	All %
Less than a year	7	19	10
1–2 years	14	10	13
3–5 years	25	38	28
5–10 years	38	26	35
More than ten years	16	8	14
Number	363	120	483

Table 3.3 Length of time that fathers had lived with the partner with whom they had a child

	Ex-married %	Ex-cohabitant %	All with a living-together relationship %
Less than a year	1	21	6
1–2 years	3	16	7
2–5 years	15	36	20
5–10 years	35	20	31
10+ years	46	7	36
Median years	9	2.5	7

Table 3.2 presents a distribution of length of time since separation, for those who had had a living-together relationship. A number of our respondents had only recently become absent fathers – 4 per cent had been absent fathers for less than six months at the time of the interview (not shown in table). The length of the episodes is determined by the constraint that our definition of non-resident fatherhood involved a child up to 16 or 18 if in full-time education. There was, as expected, a relationship between the length of time of non-resident fathering and the marital status at the time the last child was born. Fathers who had been cohabiting tended to have had the shortest periods as non-resident fathers.

Overall 10 per cent of fathers in the sample had never lived with the mother of their youngest absent child. Of those who had lived with the mother at the birth of the first non-resident child, 6 per cent had lived with her for less than a year and 36 per cent for more than ten years. As can be seen in Table 3.3 there was an association between the length of

Table 3.4 Length of time father had lived with his youngest or only
non-resident child

Length of time	%
Never lived with child	14.7
Less than one year	21.7
1–2 years	10.4
2–5 years	29.8
5–10 years	19.8
10 years or more	3.6
All (n = 535)	100

time the father had lived with the mother and marital status – ex-
cohabitants had lived with the partner for an average of 2.5 years,
compared with 9 years for the ex-married. This distribution of lengths
of living-together relationship is very similar to that for lone parents
reported by Bradshaw and Millar (1991) – in that study the median
length of marriages was 7.6 years and cohabitations 3 years, 7 years
overall.

Although 10 per cent of the fathers had never lived with the mother
of their youngest non-resident child, some 15 per cent in total had
never lived with those children (Table 3.4). This includes those fathers
who had never lived with the mother (10 per cent) and those who had
lived with her, but the relationship had ended before the child was
born. A further 22 per cent of fathers had lived with their youngest
non-resident children for less than a year and 23 per cent for at least
five years.

Becoming a single unmarried non-resident father

As we have seen, 10 per cent of the sample were single and had not
lived with the mother of their first non-resident child. Many of them
were very young, over a third (36 per cent) were under 20 when the
child was born, and many of the mothers of the children were young –
52 per cent were under 20. The majority (74 per cent) of these single
men had only one absent child (not shown).

Becoming a non-resident father as a result of
a cohabitation breakdown

Cohabitation breakdown is now the fastest-growing source of new lone
parent families (Marsh and McKay, 1993) and nearly a quarter of the

men were living in a cohabiting relationship when they became a non-resident father. These fathers tended to be slightly older on average at the birth of the first non-resident child than the single men. But 19 per cent were under 20 when they first became fathers, and 34 per cent of their partners were under 20. Again the majority of these men had only one absent child. The average length of time the fathers had cohabited before the birth of the child was twenty-five months and the average time afterwards was seventeen months.

It is possible to distinguish between three types of cohabiting relationship. First there were those that were marriage-like when they broke down: their living-together relationship had preceded the birth of the first child by at least one year, and had continued for a year or more following the child's birth (25 per cent). Of these, 44 per cent had spent over three years with their child in the mother's household. Second, in contrast 20 per cent of cohabitants had had very short relationships with the mother, living together for less than a year before the birth and separating within a year after the birth. These cohabitations may have been associated with the pregnancy, and there was little opportunity in them for a lasting relationship to have been established with their child. Finally, other cohabitations were more difficult to categorise – those that had lasted for longer than a year before the birth but ended within a year of the birth (15 per cent of all), or those that had lasted less than a year before the birth but had gone on for over a year after the birth (39 per cent).

Becoming a non-resident father as a result of the breakdown of a marriage

Ex-married fathers were still the largest group of non-resident fathers. They have the largest average number of non-resident children. The average age of the child at separation was 4 years and the average length of time that fathers had lived with the mother before the birth of the child was four years and two months – so on average these relationships had lasted over eight years. They had lived with the children for the longest period of time and, as we shall see, they are most likely still to be in contact with them. They tended to be older than the other two groups when they had their first child – only 11 per cent were under 20, and 23 per cent of their partners were under 20. However, some of these marriages had been of fairly short duration – 16 per cent of the ex-married fathers had lived with their wives for less than a year before the birth of the child, and 17 per cent had separated within a year of the birth of the child.

Table 3.5 Reasons for the breakdown of a living-together relationship

Reasons	% of fathers giving only one reason	% of fathers giving reason	% of reasons given
Partner found someone else/adultery/infidelity	34	34	25
Rowing a lot	20	31	23
Lack of communication/did not talk	20	30	21
Money or financial problems	6	12	9
You found someone else/adultery/infidelity	11	12	8
You did not give enough time to the family	(6)	4	3
Partner did not give enough time to the family	(4)	3	2
Unsatisfactory sexual relationship	(1)	4	3
Drugs/alcohol/addiction	(1)	2	(10)
Violence	(2)	2	(8)
Was more beneficial financially	(6)	2	(10)
Mental illness	(4)	2	(9)
Homosexual/lesbian	(2)	1	(3)
Number	270	441	612

Excluding other and don't knows.
Figures in brackets are numbers.

Reasons for becoming a non-resident father

Those fathers who had ever had a living-together relationship with the mother of their non-resident child were asked to give the reasons why their relationship had broken down. The results are summarised in Table 3.5. Obviously the reasons why relationships end are complex, vary over time, interact and are difficult to summarise in response to a structured questionnaire (and one that enabled the respondent to give only two reasons). Further, 29 per cent of respondents mentioned a reason other than those offered to them. If these are excluded, the most common single reason given by the fathers was that *their partner* found someone else/committed adultery/was unfaithful. This was the reason given by a third of the fathers. The next most common reason mentioned overall, was that the couple had been rowing a lot, followed by lack of communication/did not talk. Money problems were mentioned in 12 per cent of cases. Adultery of the father was only admitted as a reason in 12 per cent of cases. It is striking that violence was mentioned as a reason in only 2 per cent of cases. Lone parents in the Bradshaw and Millar (1991) study mentioned violence as a reason for the breakup in 20 per cent of cases, and as the main reason for the breakup in 13 per cent of cases. Clearly there may have been a reluctance on behalf of these fathers to acknowledge or admit violent behaviour.

Of the fathers who had been married, 83 per cent had obtained a divorce by the time of the interview. The grounds for the divorce in these cases are summarised in Table 3.6. Adultery and unreasonable behaviour were most commonly given as the grounds for divorce. In the Bradshaw and Millar (1991) study of lone parents, unreasonable behaviour was cited as the most common reason for divorce, though at that time irretrievable breakdown was not an option. Of those ex-married who had not yet been divorced, 51 per cent intended to obtain a divorce in the future.

Table 3.6 Grounds for divorce

	%
Adultery	31
Unreasonable behaviour	30
Two years' separation	12
Five years' separation	2
Desertion	1
Irretrievable breakdown (not specified)	21
Other/don't know	2
Number	329

Table 3.7 Feelings about the end of the relationship

	Ex-married %	Ex-cohabitant %
Happy	62	62
Unhappy	29	24
Neither	9	10
Don't know	1	3
Number	388	135

Table 3.8 Feelings about the breakup of the living-together relationship

	Ex-married %	Ex-cohabiting %	All %	Lone mothers* %
I'm glad I did not stay with my partner	57	61	58	57
I am glad my partner left	10	9	10	20
I did not have a say in the breakup from my partner	16	15	16	8
I wish my partner had stayed with me	6	4	6	5
I wish I had stayed with my partner	6	5	5	4
Not applicable	(5)	(2)	(7)	2
Don't know	4	5	4	6
Number	409	145	554	827

* Bradshaw and Millar, 1991.
Figures in brackets are numbers.

Overall, 62 per cent of the fathers expressed themselves happy that their living-together relationship had come to an end, and it can be seen in Table 3.7 that there was little difference between the ex-married and ex-cohabitants.

The fathers were asked about their present feelings about the breakup of their relationship, using a similar question to one employed by Bradshaw and Millar (1991), and the results are summarised in Table 3.8. Very few fathers regretted the breakup of their relationship. Only 5 per cent wished that they had stayed with their partner, and 6 per cent wished that their partner had stayed with them, whereas 58 per cent were glad that they had not stayed with their partner, and 10 per cent that their partner had not stayed with them. Compared with the lone mothers in the Bradshaw and Millar (1991) study, the main difference was that a much higher proportion of these fathers said that they had no say in the breakup of their relationship. This suggests that while they may or may not have regretted the end of their relationships, they felt that they were (passive) victims of a decision made by the mother of their children.

FINDINGS FROM THE QUALITATIVE STUDY

In this section we turn from the survey results and present some of the findings from the qualitative study on contact, which have a bearing on becoming a non-resident father. We focus on three issues in particular – the causes of the relationship breakdown, what the fathers felt about their partners at the time of breakup and the impact of work and money problems on the relationship with their former partner.

Causes of the relationship breakdown

Table 3.9 is a very simplified summary of the causes of relationship breakdown for the men in the qualitative study on contact. Life is of course a good deal messier than these simple explanations. In most cases the partnership dragged on unhappily for some time before one of the couple decided to end it. The time during which the partnership was in crisis is given in the table. Although adultery does feature as a reason for ending relationships, adultery seems to act as a catalyst rather than the cause of breakup.

As can be seen from Table 3.9 the separation was initiated in twelve cases by the mother and in eight by the father. In all but the case where the couple were not married, the decision to end the relationship came after years of difficulties. Two of the couples had been to Relate counselling to try to save the marriage, but the counselling had failed. In the case of three couples the child was born before the woman was aged 20. One young father said:

> basically I was only thinking of meself at that time. I love me children you know what I mean but I was only young 23, you know what I mean. I just felt that I should take care of meself in me own selfish way.

How fathers felt about their partner at the time of the breakup

Except for the eight fathers who had chosen to end the relationship, a common theme reiterated by the remaining fathers was their

Table 3.9 Reasons given by fathers for relationship breakdown

Case no.	Main problems	Catalyst	Time-scale	Who initiated
1	Father had been unemployed for 5 years – went to university became involved in student life	Mother suspected him of having affair – affair denied	1 year	Mother
2	Mother got evening job in club, never home; no physical relationship	Mother had affair; father found out; father had affair	2 years	Mother
3	Very young couple lived together for 3 months, father thought it worked quite well	Mother found out she was pregnant; returned to her parents	6 months	Mother
4	Mother had psychological problems, 'treated children badly', 'violent'; 'difficult' relationship	Mother had affair 10 years before, had 2nd affair	10 years	Father
5	Mother (2nd wife) got pregnant 6 weeks after they met, difficult relationship, she insecure; jealous; father's expectations high after 1st wife (who left him)	Father had affair with old girlfriend – moved in with her	2.5 years	Father
6	Both very young – 20/18; mother felt resentful at being cooped up with child	Mother left	18 months	Mother
7	Mother had many affairs, father not worried about that (gay)	Mother accused father of abusing daughter	5 years	Mother
8	Cold relationship; no intimacy or physical relationship, tried Relate	Father left – later he found out mother had been having affair for 2 years	2 years	Father
9	Father too involved in work, never home, mother fed up with being at home with 2 little kids	Mother moved away to university with the children – had affair	3 years	Mother
10	Mother became depressed after birth of child; different values, wife anti-materialistic; arguments	A new carpet	4 years	Mother

11	Mother 'neglected' 3 children; mother/child relationship difficult	Mother had affair; relationship drifted on for 2 years; after that father unable to cope	2 years	Father
12	Father became manic depressive – they had 4 children, he was 40; unable to work	Crashed the car and sectioned under the Mental Health Act	4 years	Mother
13	Incompatible personalities; 'violent, vicious' mother; difficulties with 2 stepchildren – stepson in prison	Mother had affair	years unspecified	Father
14	Mother ill, diabetes; only got married because mother pregnant; a mistake on his part; getting on each other's nerves: tried Relate, did not improve	All her friends getting divorced; no real catalyst	11 years	Father
15	Didn't do much together (shift work), money problems; had separate lives	No real catalyst	years unspecified	Mother
16	Stifling relationship; different values and expectations, father worked in evenings to avoid mother; mother involved with friends	Both had affairs	years unspecified	Father
17	Young – he was 18 she was 16; she was pregnant	Father resentful at losing youth	6 months	Father
18	Tensions in marriage, came to a head when they were living in a tied house; surrounded by his work on a farm; mother hated it	Mother moved out without telling him	1 year	Mother
19	Money and different attitudes and personality; went to work abroad to clear debts	Mother decided to leave him while he was abroad	4 years	Mother
20	Had three heart attacks	Mother returned to ex-husband	1 year	Mother

'victimisation'. The fathers felt victimised and outraged by their partners, and frequently asked themselves what they had done to deserve this treatment. The three men who were the most bitter, and remained bitter after many years, were the fathers whose wives had left them without any warning. One man who had been working abroad in India for two years received a letter from his wife telling him not to come home anymore, because she wanted a divorce. He maintained he did not know that there were any problems in the relationship.

> Well she'd obviously . . . was waiting for the opportunity to make the break well before that from what I gather. Well she wanted, she said she wanted to leave before [daughter] was born, cos we moved house and she found she was pregnant again, so she just lumped it again and that's what she said 'I'm only staying for the girls at the moment', and you know, I said 'Well what am I doing wrong?' She said, 'Nothing, it's what you didn't do.' I said, 'Well what am I meant to do?' And I just, she just said 'Rubbish you know, stupid things'. . . . I've always got a long face when I go shopping, you know, like every husband has, you know. It's just stupid things like that.

A large distance between the fathers and their children following separation was a compounding factor adding to the bitterness. Another of the three fathers whose wives had left without warning, was even more distressed the following year when she and his children moved again, 500 miles away, without telling him. That was five years ago and he is still bitter, and unable to form a new relationship. The most angry and bitter of the three men was the politics student whose wife left him, taking the children, and returned to her home town 250 miles away.

> I knew she was unhappy from September. Then in December she told me that she had phoned her brother up and he was coming to fetch her. And that was the first I knew that she was going to leave. She then said it was just for a bit and she might come back. But she never did, she never did come back. . . . I was very unhappy, very unhappy. No doctor, no counselling, still doing my degree another year and a half. There were two tutors I talked to. . . . We had a law department and I saw a gentleman there who told me the best way of doing things – but that was several months after. I never thought it would come to that. The following October I was divorced and I didn't even know. In November I got a letter that said there was going to be a case to sort out access to the children

and I went down there, and the law department had assured me that this would be sorted out before any divorce and when I went down I had been divorced for a month and didn't know. I was expecting to be still married.

This is how the man summed up his feelings at the time:

At that time I think I hated her, in fact I know I did. I think if I could have I'd have killed her.

For the other eight men, who decided to leave the relationship, all commented on the fact that the decision had been difficult to make, for numerous reasons. Even so, the separation was the most difficult, painful event that had ever happened to any of them. One of the men who left said he could not survive in the emotionally and physically cold environment of his marriage, he did not know his wife had been having an affair until after he left. They had tried going to Relate, which had failed, and he had stopped trying to save the relationship. When he found out the real reason for his wife's coldness, he was angry and depressed and felt that he had been taken for a fool.

Working wives/partners

Many men would have preferred their partners to stay at home and look after the family. Yet only three of the ex-partners had not been working during the time they had lived together. In all of these cases the children were very young and it would have been extremely difficult for the partner to contemplate a job in the circumstances. All the women worked part-time, most only working for a few hours a day. All the women had insecure positions and most, apart from the part-time free-lance journalist and teacher, were badly paid. A list of occupations includes: a waitress, two cleaners, two shop assistants, three office workers, a plasterer, a student, a bar maid and a home worker.

Some women wanted to work out of choice. Paul reported that his wife could not bear staying at home with just a small baby for company, while he worked his long hours. She was not socialised to expect to stay home and keep house, she was a young energetic woman and she wanted her own world, and friends and money.

When my wife gave birth to Simon I said 'You are not working full stop.' When he was about 6 weeks − 8 weeks she gave up breast feeding anyway. She picked him up one evening and said 'I want to go back to work. I just can't cope.' I said 'What do you want to do?' And she said 'Perhaps something one night a week'; and I regret letting her go . . . because I'm not inferring anything about her motherhood . . . but that's the first time I realised she was a career woman.

Effects of working long hours on relationships

All of the sample, talking retrospectively with the experience of hindsight, were aware of how much their absence at work, the long hours they had put in, had contributed to the deterioration of their relationship with their ex-partner. They had felt this conflict between work and home and five of the fathers felt that their commitment to their jobs had been a major factor in their problems with their ex-wives. They could see, looking back, where they had gone wrong in leaving their partners alone, neglecting them in subtle ways, but had felt at the time that they were under pressure to provide, and there was no alternative choice.

The loneliness of the young mothers, coping with young children constantly, was mentioned time and again. It was the major cause of at least one divorce. As a result of Henry's commitment to his job as a financial adviser, which took him out of the house visiting clients in the daytime, in the evening and also at weekends, his wife, Sara, felt neglected. He said she decided she wanted a career of her own and went to university to do a degree. By the second term her view of the world had completely changed, she had recovered her bruised self-esteem, found a new boyfriend and decided to leave Henry. Henry had the insight to see that his behaviour had been the root cause of the problem and that Sara and the children needed his time and attention. He tried desperately to keep the marriage together, and promised to change and become more involved with her and the children, but it was too late.

> I suppose largely, um . . . Me getting involved with organisations and committees which took time away from me actually putting the family first . . . um, and as a result her feeling that I didn't really love her that much any more . . . and certainly put other things before giving commitment of time and weekends for her and the children.
> [Long pause, before he continues.]
> She had some sort of flu, viral infection and was err feeling really run down, looking after two, young, very small kids as well. . . . I mean hindsight is a wonderful thing as it often is . . . um, I cannot believe that I actually did that. That I actually went off to London to a committee meeting. Not only that but stayed overnight and

instead of coming back and missed the train on Saturday, so I didn't wander back until one, or two on Saturday afternoon . . . er just probably selfish really . . . or blinkered. I mean looking back on it, I wasn't aware of how . . . tunnelled vision I'd become.

One of the fathers on incapacity benefit had been a long-distance lorry driver who was away three or four nights every week, leaving his wife to manage a part-time job and four young children alone. He felt that this was one of the contributing factors to his problems.

Well I spoke to her and said if you want me to take a different job where I'm at home every night just say so. . . . Which I tried. She said to me 'I'll give you 6 months before you're back on the road driving.' She was right. She said I was unreasonable and I suppose I was in some respects.

Money problems

However easy or difficult it was to manage the long work hours, the men said they were usually driven to work overtime out of necessity and the need for money. Money problems were a common theme associated with the breadwinner role, both during the relationship and at the end of the relationship. Table 3.10 summarises the men's primary reaction to money problems and the final settlement that was made. Only four of the fathers had come out of the relationship with what they felt was a reasonable financial deal. Two of these fathers had managed this because they had financial acumen – one was a financial adviser and the other father had negotiated a deal at the height of the property boom. He had bought his wife out, arranged a maintenance agreement, then had sold the marital home at a profit. The third man had a wife who was 'obsessively anti-materialistic' and would only accept a share of the home, and a fourth man had a high-earner wife. Seven of the fathers lost the owner occupier status they had achieved while in the partnership and only one has since been able to take on another mortgage five years after his divorce.

Sorting out the financial assets at the end of the relationship was a difficult task, especially on top of the property settlements (if any) and the child maintenance; some claimed to have huge debts, as they picked up the bills in the aftermath of their relationships. The nature of the debts meant that many men were paying weekly hire-purchase agreements on furniture that they would not have the use of and this was a cause for anger and bitterness.

Table 3.10 Money problems

Case no.	Mortgage during partnership	Mortgage after partnership	Debts	Circumstances now	Attitude to ex-partner
1	No, council house	Bought council house	Yes	Poor, as no house during marriage, all money goes on children	Bitter
2	Yes, had bought a house on mortgage before marriage	Lost house, now in council house	Yes, £20,000 hire-purchase	Went bankrupt; struggling to get back to his former affluence	Bitter
3	No	No, living with parents	Yes	No	Bitter
4	Yes	Yes, made money on boom	Yes	Made money on sale of house at time of property boom	OK; glad it happened
5	Yes	Lost house after 5 years, has mortgage	Yes	Paying 20% of income to second wife and 1 child (has 4 other children)	Very bitter
6	No	Mortgage after marriage over	Yes	Pays through CSA	Gets on OK
7	No	No	Yes	Has no assets	Still loves wife
8	Mortgage	Mortgage	Yes	High-earner wife, split property	OK
9	Mortgage	Mortgage	Yes	Living in house with lodger, wife accusing him of hiding resources	OK – wife bitter
10	Mortgage	Mortgage	No	Wife anti-materialistic; had a split of property, no maintenance	OK
11	Mortgage	Lost house, council house	Yes	Made redundant; out of work 18 months	Bitter

12	Mortgage	Lost house, lives with mother	Yes	Manic-depressive; on benefit; poor	Bitter
13	Mortgage	Lost house, lives with brothers	Yes	Chronic sick; waiting compensation from car crash	Bitter
14	Council house	Council house – low pay	Yes	Low pay; no assets	OK
15	Mortgage	Lost house, living with parents	Yes	CSA arrears	Bitter
16	Mortgage	Mortgage	Yes	CSA arrears; wife also bitter	Bitter
17	No mortgage	Mortgage years later	Yes	Young at time, no assets, wife bitter	OK
18	Mortgage	Mortgage	Yes	Wife moved 500 miles away, makes visiting difficult and expensive – money for public school	Bitter
19	Mortgage	Mortgage on low pay	Yes, huge debts	Worked abroad because of debts; low pay now, CSA assessment lower than he was paying	Very bitter
20	Mortgage	Lost house, council house	Yes	3 heart attacks, lost job, wife left, lost house	OK

I had just bought new central heating, ere, and I had all new furniture while I'd been in there – on that buy now, pay later . . . an she knew it was all due to be paid in January; the whole lot paid out in January, nearly £2,000 . . . an there was a gas fire, cooker and all that . . . an I paid it off . . . you know January and February . . . now come to March she put straight in for a divorce . . . an she wasn't daft. She knew it all had to be paid out in January. She got the lot. The house, all I got was a bed, a wardrobe and a sideboard . . . an she got the house, the furniture, the cooker, the washer, the dryer; the new gas fires, everything . . . cos I'd put in new gas fires as well with a new back boiler . . . new sofas . . . new chairs.

It was worse when the ex-partner sold off the assets that were still being paid for on hire-purchase.

I told the solicitor she's changed the locks and my name was still on the mortgage . . . now I couldn't get into my own house . . . by then she had started selling off stuff . . . there was some stuff that was on hire-purchase which she should not have sold because it didn't belong to her . . . but I went to the hire-purchase company and said . . . 'look . . . it's still on hire-purchase . . . I can't get the goods out of the house, she's got them . . . what do I do?' They say 'Oh well; you'll have to pay for it' . . . and I says 'Oh no'; so . . . which I thought was not fair cos if I'd got the goods . . . or she'd took over the payments fair enough . . . but it ended up on me. By the time I was finished with it all there was about twenty grand debt. I ended up getting bankrupt because of it. I was homeless . . . nowhere to go . . . I made me self bankrupt. It was much easier.

The men who were the most bitter at the end of their relationships were those who had struggled for many years on low pay, had managed to buy a house on a mortgage and then had lost their home.

I lost everything. You see I had bought that house [on a mortgage] before I met her. Me mam and dad were very upset about it. You see I had worked all that time and never ended up with nothing.

The strong feelings that this loss incurs sometimes run over into the relationship with children.

There is, I mean, there is considerable residual resentment in me, which I have to overcome to, you know, treat James, well you know and fairly and all the rest of it. But every penny of capital I've laid out on the house – for more than 20 years has disappeared and that was that. But I do feel a considerable amount of resentment at the moment towards him [son]. There are times when I am quite bad tempered and I actually find him quite irritating. The only child very over protected by a sort of very, very obsessive mother and positively adored, loved an spoiled – but I find him a tiresome, spoilt child.

Most of the men in this sample thought they had a raw deal in terms of losing their homes and their children. In the next chapter we will deal in greater depth with the emotional sense of 'loss' these fathers experienced. Here we concentrate on the financial problems affecting these fathers as they battled with the depression all of them, whatever the circumstances, claimed to have endured. One theme that came through again and again was that these fathers did not know what they had done wrong; they had tried to be good husbands and good fathers.

Relationship breakdown and employment

We investigated the employment pattern at the time of the marriage breakdown to see how marriage breakdown might affect the fathers' employment. We asked the men to talk about how they had felt about their jobs at the time of separation, and if there had been any changes in their working patterns at this time. All the men had a different story to tell, and there were individual differences in the way they reacted to stress; but there were many similarities. They all admitted to being 'off course' and 'slightly deranged' for a few months. At the time of the separation all the men found that it was difficult to concentrate and focus their attention on their jobs and they felt that their work performance had suffered. The self-employed financial adviser lost business and money and his problems were exacerbated by the fact that he had moved to another town to be near his wife, who had gone off to start a university degree. For all the sample, we found it was a time of great internal and external change, but nine of the men remained in the same job right through their marriage breakdown. Four of the men were professionals in secure jobs, but another five of the men were in an assortment of manual and clerical jobs. Three men changed their jobs at this time. One man changed his job but remained in the same company – he stopped working abroad and came back to England; one man decided to risk all when there was no restraint on how he managed his life and became self-employed. Three men gave up their jobs very soon after their separation. One young man gave up his job because he was only paid on commission, and he decided that he did not like this sort of pressure on his life, or the job he was doing. He was unemployed, living at home with his own parents (where he still is), for three months and then he got a job with the local authority where he has been working for the past four years. The two other men went abroad – for different reasons. One man who had declared himself bankrupt went off to a Greek island where he became a waiter for a season; and the other man, Terry, went to the south of France where he also worked at a seasonal job. (Both these men came back and resumed their relationships with their families.) The experience of work and unemployment for one of the men and the relationship between the two went in the opposite direction to that we had hypothesised. He lived in the Midlands, and had been long-term unemployed for five years since his redundancy. Even though they had no money, he said he and his wife had been very happy together, doing everything together and sharing responsibilities for the children. He said in thirteen years he and his wife never argued. At the age of 35, he decided to take a politics degree, as a way out of unemployment. As he became more engrossed in his new world, his wife became more alienated from him. She became suspicious of his activities and friends and decided to leave him. He got his degree, he got a job as a civil servant, but in the meantime he lost his marriage. In retrospect, he said he wished he had stayed long-term unemployed; he was happier married than he has been since with a degree and his civil service job.

The three men on incapacity benefit had all lost their health, their jobs and their marriages. Their lives had changed beyond all recognition from the lives they had lived with their partners, although none of them were depressed or bitter at the time of interview. The HGV driver's second marriage had ended finally, when he had suffered three very severe heart attacks and was told he could never work again. He had his driving licence taken from him. For a while he became a 'couch potato' and was unable to do anything, again putting more pressure on his wife and young children – they still had three children under the age of ten. The ending of his marriage at this stage he saw as a major contradiction in the behaviour of his wife, who had always wanted him to be more at home. She now had him at home full-time, but instead of being able to take joint care of the home and the children, and do things with her, he was an invalid. Their standard of living was much reduced, as they now lived on incapacity benefit. His wife felt she had had as much as she could take with this relationship and solved the problem by returning to her first husband. The father was resigned, but went on to make a new life for himself, and another relationship.

A similar fate awaited a father who suffered from manic depression. His wife left him two years after he had been diagnosed manic-depressive. In the early stages of his illness, he had been unable to accept his diagnosis and refused to take medication. Before starting his medication he was compulsorily admitted to psychiatric hospital eight times. His wife left him because she could not cope with the madness that surrounded him, and it was many years before he was able to see his children again.

CHARACTERISTICS OF NON-RESIDENT FATHERS

In this section we return to the survey results and examine the present circumstances of the non-resident fathers. Table 3.11 summarises some of the key circumstances of the fathers in the study at the time of the interview, and where possible these characteristics are compared with those households (or benefit units where appropriate) where there was a father with a resident child, using data derived from an analysis of the Family Resources Survey (FRS) 1994/95. The fathers in the FRS included a small number of resident fathers (2.8 per cent) who as well as having a resident child were paying child support/maintenance to another household. Most of these were paying in respect of a child – only 11 out of 175 were paying maintenance in respect of a former partner and not a child. Also included are men who are resident fathers or stepfathers and who may also be non-resident fathers but are not paying child support. However, the FRS sample of fathers does not include (because they cannot be identified) non-resident fathers who have no children living with them. We found 3 per cent of men in the FRS aged 16–65, with no children living in their household, who were paying maintenance/child support.

Just over a third (36 per cent) of the fathers in this survey were living alone at the time of the interview and 42 per cent were living with a new partner. Among the rest, 4 per cent were living with some of their own children, but not with female partners; therefore some of these non-resident fathers were also lone parents to some of their children and some had shared care of their children who happened to be resident at the time of the interview. Five per cent of fathers were living with their children from a previous relationship only. However, a further 6 per cent had children living with them from a mix of relationships, that is combinations of children from previous relationships alongside stepchildren and/or new children.

Table 3.11 Current circumstances of non-resident fathers

	Non-resident fathers %	All resident fathers in the FRS 1994/95 %
Household composition		
living alone	36	—
living with a partner only	16	—
living with a partner and children	26	97
living with children only	4	3
living with relatives (no partner or child)	9	—
other	9	—
Current marital status		
married	18	90.2
living as married	27	7.6
single	8	0.5
married but separated	23	0.6
divorced	25	1.1
widowed	—	0.4
Present partner	57 per cent or 338 have no partner	Not available
married to you	58	
single never married	21	
divorced	17	
widowed	(1)	
still married to someone else	3	
Children		Not available
no child in the household	70	
new children only	11	
child from father's previous relationship only	5	
stepchild only	9	
a mixture of children	6	
Number of children in the household		
0	70	—
1	15	37.5
2	9	43.6
3	4	14.5
4	1	3.4
5	(1)	0.7
6	(1)	0.5
Number of dependent children outside the household		Not available
1	53	
2	36	
3	8	
4	2	
5	(3)	
6	(1)	

Table 3.11 (cont'd)

	Non-resident fathers %	All resident fathers in the FRS 1994/95 %
Number of dependent children inside and outside the household		Not available
1	38	
2	34	
3	16	
4	7	
5	3	
6	2	
7	(3)	
8	(2)	
Number of people in the household		
1	36	—
2	25	1.3
3	17	29.0
4	14	46.3
5+	7	23.4
Age of youngest child in the household		
0–4	48	44
5–10	33	28
11–18	19	28
Age of youngest dependent child outside the household		Not available
0–4	21	
5–10	45	
11–18	35	
Father's age		
under 25	5	2.7
25–30	14	14.1
31–34	25	17.0
35–40	23	26.6
41–49	28	30.0
50+	5	9.6
Ethnic group		
white	95	93
black Caribbean	3	0.7
black African	1	0.4
black other	1	0.1
Asian	(1)	4.5
other	(3)	1.1
Social class (omnibus)		
professional and intermediate	19	27
skilled non-manual	17	18
skilled manual	30	38
partly skilled manual	19	14
unskilled manual	15	5

Table 3.11 (cont'd)

	Non-resident fathers %	All resident fathers in the FRS 1994/95 %
Age finished full-time schooling (omnibus)		
under 14	3	2.8
15	24	21.5
16	44	40.7
17–18	14	16.4
19+	16	18.6
still at school	2	—
Qualifications		Not available
none	32	
CSE/GCE/GCSE/School Certificate	55	
Ordinary National Certificate or Diploma	10	
BTech/A level/Scottish Higher	15	
Higher National Certificate or Diploma	10	
Degree	6	
Postgraduate	2	
any other	15	
Vocational qualifications		
apprenticeship	23	Not available
City and Guilds	30	
clerical commercial computer related	9	
nursing	1	
teaching	4	
professional (accountancy, law, insurance, etc.)	6	
armed forces	10	
social work	1	
any other	10	
none	41	
Do you have a long-term illness or disability which limits your daily activities?		
yes	20	14
no	80	86
How would you rate your health generally compared to the people of your age?		Not available
excellent	15	
good	51	
fair	25	
poor	7	
very poor	2	

Figures in brackets are numbers.

Of the 42 per cent of fathers who had a new partner, just over half (58 per cent) were married to that partner. Of the fathers living in new partnerships, 60 per cent contained children and nearly a third of these (31 per cent) contained the partner's children from a previous relationship (not shown). Thus 19 per cent of the non-resident fathers in this sample who had repartnered, had repartnered with women who were lone mothers.[9] This is a highly significant finding because one of the best routes out of poverty for lone mothers is to repartner, and in a marriage market where men tend to partner younger women, it is inevitable that the new potential partners for lone mothers will tend to be men who may have already been in child-bearing partnerships.

In total, taking those fathers with new children only and a mixture of children only, 17 per cent of the fathers had had new children in a new partnership. Of those households with new children 11 per cent (sixty-eight) had one child and a further 4 per cent (twenty-three) had two children (not shown). However, if account is taken of the number of dependent children inside and outside the household non-resident fathers are more likely than resident fathers to have had three or more. This is the result of a combination of children brought to and born to the new relationship.

Non-resident fathers' households are smaller than all fathers, and the children in the households tend to be younger than resident fathers' children. Though the non-resident children tend to be older, non-resident fathers themselves are younger than fathers in general.

Only 5 per cent of the fathers in the sample were non-white and almost all of these were black. Although it is difficult to be certain from such a small subsample, it is probable from our results and studies of lone mothers, that non-resident fathers are more likely to be black Caribbean and less likely to be Asian than resident fathers.

The subject of employment is dealt with in detail in Chapter 4, but it is clear from the comparisons in this table that non-resident fathers are less likely than resident fathers to be in social class 1 and more likely to be in social class 5. They are also more likely to have left school at younger ages and (although there is no comparison data) appear to have low academic or vocational qualifications. They are also more likely than fathers in general to have a long-term illness or disability – only 15 per cent describe their health as excellent and 9 per cent describe it as poor or very poor.

As will be seen in Chapter 4 these characteristics have a knock-on effect on their employment and income and in Chapter 8 it will be seen to have an effect on their capacity to pay child support.

Table 3.12 Fathers' family of origin and relationships with them

	Non-resident fathers (%)
Childhood	
lived with both parents	73
lived with natural mother only	9
lived with natural father only	2
lived with natural mother and stepfather	6
lived with natural father and stepmother	2
lived with grandparents	3
adopted	2
lived with foster parents	1
spent time in care	2
If lone mother was she (n = 93)	
widowed	20
divorce/separated	73
single lone mother	8
Father's occupation	
professional/technical	13
higher administrative	5
clerical	4
sales	3
service	6
skilled worker	38
semi-skilled worker	18
unskilled worker	12
farm	2
How often do you see members of your parental family?	
at least once a week	60
at least once a fortnight	6
at least once a month	9
at least every three months	6
once or twice a year	6
less often	4
not at all	8
Nearest parental family member within 10 miles	
none	30
parent	60
sibling/grandparent	38
other	11

Fathers' family of origin

We were interested to collect some data about the fathers' family of origin, in order to establish their family and class background and their present relationships with their families. It can be seen in Table 3.12 that 27 per cent of these men had not lived with both their natural parents throughout their childhood. Among these, 15 per cent had spent time with their mothers, 4 per cent with their fathers and 5 per cent had experienced adoption, fostering or time in care. There are no data that enable us to see how this compares with all fathers, and the proportion with an experience of family disruption is certainly less than the present generation of children will experience. However, the proportion of fathers with experience of care looks high. The social class classification of the fathers of these non-resident fathers indicates that they are much more likely to come from working-class families.

The fathers still appeared to have close relationships with their family of origin. Only 8 per cent had no contact, 60 per cent saw members of their parental family at least once a week and 75 per cent at least once a month. Only 30 per cent had no parental family member living within ten miles.

In the qualitative study we also investigated how important the father's extended family was in helping him to maintain contact with his children and these results will be discussed in Chapter 7.

SUMMARY

In this chapter we have presented some evidence, from the survey and one of the qualitative studies, on the process of becoming a non-resident father. The experience of separation and divorce is almost invariably a painful process. Although there were few fathers who now regretted the end of their relationship, how the breakdown occurred, who they thought was responsible for it, and the extent to which they felt they had any control over events, will have had a lasting impact on the relationship with their ex-partner and their children. Another factor affecting these relationships is the length of time that they lasted, and particularly whether the parents were living together with their child long enough to have established a bond.

The characteristics of the non-resident fathers have shown that they tend to be in lower social class groups, to be younger, to live in smaller households, and to have poorer health than fathers in general. Although non-resident fathers tended to live in smaller households as over a third were living alone, nearly half were living with a new partner and the majority of those had children living in their households and were married to their new partners. The majority also lived close to their families of origin (parents and siblings) and saw them at least weekly, suggesting a stable life-style.

4 Employment and income

INTRODUCTION

The analysis in Chapter 2 revealed that even after the sample was reweighted only two-thirds of non-resident fathers were in employment. This is a much lower proportion than would be expected of a general sample of fathers – 84 per cent of fathers in the Family Resources Survey 1994/95 were in employment. This low level of labour participation has important consequences for the incomes and living standards of these men. It may be both a cause and consequence of their being non-resident fathers and it certainly has implications for their capacity to contribute towards child support and their chances of forming new families. Employment and income are therefore the subjects of this chapter. Here we draw exclusively on the findings from the sample survey of the non-resident fathers.[10]

EMPLOYMENT

Two-thirds (66 per cent) of the fathers had had a paid job in the past seven days but not all of the others were unemployed (using the International Labour Office definition). Of those not in paid employment, only about half (52 per cent) were looking for work in the past four weeks, and 6 per cent of those said that they would not have been able to start work if a job had been available. So the actual unemployment rate among these fathers was 17 per cent – still much higher than the 9 per cent unemployment rate found among all fathers in the FRS using a similar definition. Of those unemployed and looking for work a fifth (20 per cent) had been unemployed for six weeks or less, over half (54 per cent) had been unemployed for six months or more, 15 per cent for over a year, and two fathers had been unemployed for five years.

Among the 16 per cent of the total sample who were unemployed but not looking for work about half (55 per cent) were unable to work due to sickness or disability, 5 per cent were in full-time education and nine fathers were looking after home and family. Five of these were living only with children and therefore were likely to be lone fathers as well as being non-resident fathers.

Types of jobs

Table 4.1 provides a classification of the types of jobs the fathers had. Given the relative risks of unemployment, it is not surprising to find that non-resident fathers in employment are much more likely to be in professional, technical or clerical jobs, whereas unemployed non-resident fathers are more likely to have worked previously in semi-skilled or unskilled jobs. It is also striking that non-resident fathers both in and outside employment are more likely to be in lower status (and on average worse-paid jobs) than fathers in general. Although the classifications are not identical, there are far fewer non-resident fathers in professional and managerial jobs and more in unskilled manual jobs.

About 13 per cent of the whole sample and 20 per cent of those in employment are self-employed. This is very similar to the proportion of

Table 4.1 Classification of the jobs of non-resident fathers compared with all fathers

	Main job of those in employment	Last job of those not in employment	All non-resident fathers	Jobs of all fathers 1994/95 Family Resources Survey
	%	%	%	%
Professional/technical	22	9	18	42
Higher administrative	4	(1)	3	10*
Clerical	5	2	3	
Sales	6	6	6	
Service	12	7	10	
Skilled worker	28	29	28	33
Semi-skilled worker	14	25	18	12
Unskilled worker	10	21	14	3
Farm	1	1	1	
Total %	100	100	100	100
Total number	384	228	579	6,288

* skilled non-manual.

fathers in the whole population who are self-employed, 15 per cent of the whole population and 18 per cent of those in employment.

Hours worked

Figure 4.1 gives a distribution of the hours worked by those in employment. Six per cent of the fathers were working part-time (less than

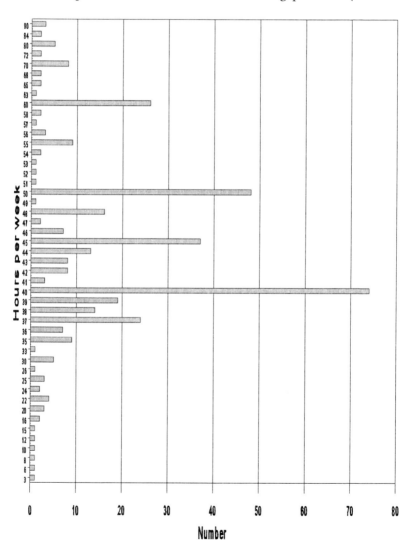

Figure 4.1 Distribution of hours worked by those in employment

30 hours per week), but over half of the fathers were working over 40 hours per week and 18 per cent were working over 50 hours a week. One might hypothesise that non-resident fathers would be employed for longer hours than fathers in general. Longer working hours might be associated with the breakdown in the relationship with their former partner, or a consequence of relationship breakdown (the absence of domestic commitments among many of these men), or they may work longer in order to recoup the resources lost at the breakdown of their relationships, or because of the extra burden of child support. However, there was no evidence to support this hypothesis – the self-employed worked an average of 51 hours per week compared with 43 hours for employees. These hours are identical to those worked by fathers in general.

Most (87 per cent) of those in employment had been in continuous employment for over a year, but 6 per cent had been in employment for less than three months. There was no difference in the lengths of employment between the self-employed and employees, but the unskilled workers had much shorter spells in employment than the other groups – 94 months compared with an average for the whole sample of 158 months.

Table 4.2 examines the odds of non-resident fathers being in employment using logistic regression. The first column presents the results of a bivariate analysis. The second column presents the results of a logistic regression with all variables forced in, and the third column presents the results of the best-fitting model, including only those variables that contribute to explaining whether the non-resident father is in employment. Some of the variables that appear to be significant in the bivariate analysis fall out in the best-fitting model, including vocational qualifications, age of the youngest non-resident child and father's age. One variable that did not appear to be significant in the bivariate analysis – the age of the youngest resident child – becomes important in the best-fitting model. The model shows that non-resident fathers are less likely to be in employment if they were cohabiting at the birth of the child, are not married now, have a resident child aged less than 10, have a long-term illness and no academic qualifications. Each of these factors is significant when all other factors have been controlled for.

Partners' employment

Among the non-resident fathers, 43 per cent had a partner living with them, and about two-thirds (65 per cent) of those partners were in employment. This is a similar rate to the partners of resident fathers in

Table 4.2 Odds of being in employment

Variable	Bivariate	Simultaneous	Best-fitting
Marital status			
single	1.00	1.00	1.00
married	2.65★★★	5.60★★★	6.02★★★
cohabiting	1.93★★	2.81★★	2.95★★
Marital status at child's birth			
single	1.09	1.81	1.80
married	2.92★★★	3.80★★★	4.09★★★
cohabiting	1.00	1.00	1.00
Age			
16–29	1.00	1.00	1.00
30–34	2.09★	1.11	1.23
35–39	3.22★★★	1.85	2.14★
40–44	1.66	0.61	0.77
45+	1.37	0.86	1.10
Age of youngest resident child			
no children	1.00	1.00	1.00
0–4	0.94	0.25★★★	0.25★★★
5–10	0.86	0.26★★	0.27★★
11–18	1.31	0.88	0.90
Age of youngest non-resident child			
0–4	1.00	1.00	
5–10	1.76★	1.34	
11–18	2.12★★	1.54	
Long-term illness or disability			
yes	1.00	1.00	1.00
no	6.29★★★	7.14★★★	7.14★★★
Academic qualifications			
none	1.00	1.00	1.00
some	2.62★★★	2.21★★★	2.36★★★
Vocational qualifications			
none	1.00	1.00	
some	1.78★★	1.33	

★$p < 0.05$; ★★$p < 0.01$; ★★★$p < 0.001$.

the FRS where 63 per cent are in employment. The distribution of partners' hours is summarised in Figure 4.2. Ten per cent were working less than 16 hours per week, but two-thirds (63 per cent) were working over 30 hours per week. This compares with 23 per cent of the partners of resident fathers working less than 16 hours per week, and 42 per cent working over 30 hours a week. Thus, this suggests that the partners of non-resident fathers are no more likely to be in employment, but if they are, they tend to work more hours. This is probably associated with the fact that they do not all have children at home.

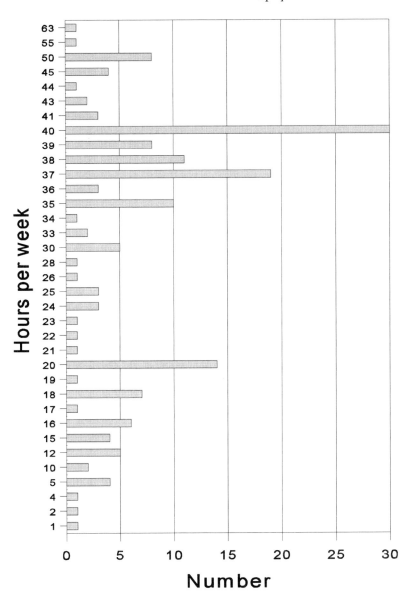

Figure 4.2 Distribution of partners' hours

Table 4.3 Type of job of the partners of non-resident fathers

	Partners of non-resident fathers %	Partners of resident fathers in the FRS %
Professional/technical	23	30
Higher administrative	4	
Clerical	28	37*
Sales	8	
Service	11	
Skilled worker	5	6
Semi-skilled worker	9	20
Unskilled worker	13	7
Total N = 163		

* skilled non-manual.

The continuity of employment among the partners was rather less than among the non-resident fathers – 15 per cent had been in their jobs for less than a year, but 70 per cent had been in their jobs for over three years.

The type of work that the partners did is summarised in Table 4.3. The partners are less likely to be skilled workers than the fathers, and more likely to be in clerical work and sales, reflecting 'female' jobs. The comparison with the FRS is complicated by the fact that the classification is not identical, but compared with the partners of fathers in general the partners of non-resident fathers appear to be less likely to be in professional and managerial jobs and more likely to be in unskilled jobs.

Table 4.4 shows that partners were much more likely to be employed if the non-resident fathers were employed. There was no variation in the employment by the age of the partners, nor by the partners' marital status. However, as would be expected, partners were much more likely to be in employment if they did not have any resident children, and much less likely if the resident child was under 5 years old.

The non-resident fathers with partners who were not in employment were asked to identify the reasons for their not working outside the home. The reasons given are summarised in Table 4.5. The most commonly mentioned reason was a general preference to be at home looking after the children; next that it was not financially worthwhile, that they could not afford child-care, and the lack of jobs in the area. Those mentioning financial incentives were examined in more detail and 59 per cent had a partner who was not in employment and therefore had some cause to claim that it was not worth working. This also ties in with the earlier

Table 4.4 Employment of the partners of non-resident fathers

	Not employed	Employed part-time	Employed full-time	Number
Non-resident father's employment				
not working but looking for work	72	13	16	32
not working/not looking for work	66	10	24	29
employed	23	5	71	188
Age of partner				
16–29	33	8	59	85
30–34	38	(2)	59	69
35–39	38	(3)	55	47
40+	31	(4)	60	48
Partner's marital status				
married to you	35	7	58	144
single never married	37	(1)	62	52
divorced	36	(2)	59	44
widowed			(1)	1
married to someone else	(1)	(2)	(5)	8
don't know/refused			(1)	1
Presence of children				
yes	47	8	45	153
no	17	25	53	100
Age of youngest resident child				
0–4	61	(4)	34	83
5–10	37	(5)	53	49
11–18	(4)	(3)	68	22

Figures in brackets are numbers.

Table 4.5 Reasons given for the partner not working

	Percentage giving reason for not working
Prefers to be at home looking after the children	48
Financially not worth it	28
Cannot afford the cost of child-care	25
Lack of jobs in the area	22
Cannot find job with convenient hours	13
Not satisfied with the quality of child-care	6
Caring for a dependent relative	5
Child-care is inconvenient	(1)
Other reason given	26

Figures in brackets are numbers.

Table 4.6 Employment of couples in the study of non-resident fathers
compared with fathers in general

	Non-resident fathers study %	Family Resources Survey %
Neither partner employed	17	12
Father and partner employed part-time	4	13
Father and partner employed full-time	56	44
Father employed and partner not employed	18	28
Father not employed and partner employed	7	4
Number	249	6,288

finding that partners are much less likely to be working if the non-resident fathers are not employed.

Table 4.6 shows how the employment of the couples in this study compares with the employment of fathers and their partners in the Family Resources Survey. Given the small numbers in the non-resident fathers sample with partners, it is necessary to be wary of drawing too firm conclusions from this comparison, but there does appear to be a higher proportion among the non-resident fathers with neither partner in employment, but a higher proportion of families where both the non-resident father and their partner are both working full-time.

INCOME

Given the findings on the employment of non-resident fathers we can expect that their incomes will be lower than fathers in general, which will have an impact on their living standards, their capacity to pay maintenance and to support a second family. In this section we explore the sources of income of the fathers and, if they have them, their partners, analyse the level of their total income, and draw conclusions about their living standards.

The results are presented both including the self-employed and excluding them. This is because of the problems of assessing self-employed incomes. In the sample 13 per cent (n = 76) were self-employed, and 58 per cent of these (n = 44) ran their own business, and drew up profit and loss accounts. We attempted to assess their incomes by taking what the net profit of their share of the business was in the previous year, or the most recent period for which they had figures. Only 57 per cent (n = 25) were able to provide an amount (which ranged from £2,000 to £170,000 per year). Four other cases said that they had made nothing, or a loss, and the rest did not know, or did not reply. The rest of the self-employed (n = 30), who worked for an organisation, or who ran their own business, but did not draw up profit and loss accounts, were asked to estimate their before tax income in the past twelve months. NOP had made a mistake in their CAPI routing for this question, and no one in their sample was asked this question so we have data for only sixteen cases, just over half this group of self-employed. For these reasons there is cause to be anxious about the accuracy of the income data for the self-employed.

However, the majority of the sample were employees, and they were asked to provide their usual gross pay, that is including any overtime, bonuses, tips, commissions and so on, before any deduction for tax, National Insurance or pension contributions, union dues and so on. Ninety-five per cent of those who were in employment were able to provide this information. They were then asked their usual take-home pay, that is after any deductions for income tax, National Insurance, union dues and pension contributions. Ninety-four per cent were able to provide this information. Employees and the self-employed were also asked to provide information on any income from a second job or odd jobs – 7 per cent provided information on other jobs. In addition 28 per cent of the sample had a partner who was earning, and 78 per cent of the fathers were able to provide an estimate of her gross earnings and 73 per cent of her net earnings.

Table 4.7 provides a summary of the weekly income of the non-resident fathers divided into its separate components. In the sections below we comment on each component of the income.

Earnings

The gross earnings of the respondents excluding the self-employed averaged £324 (sd = 191) and ranged from £17 to £1,481 per week. Net earnings ranged from £17 to £969 per week. Figure 4.3 gives a frequency distribution of the hourly rates of pay for respondents. The mean hourly rate of the fathers was £7 (sd = 4) (compared with an hourly rate of £9.68 for resident fathers) but 7 per cent were working for less than £3 per hour. The net pay of partners averaged £136 (sd = 77) per week and the distribution of their hourly rates of pay is shown in Figure 4.4. The mean hourly rate was £5.76 per hour (sd = 3) (compared with an hourly rate of £5.98 for the partners of resident fathers) but nearly a quarter were working for £3 per hour or less.

Table 4.7 Income data

	Including the self-employed			Excluding the self-employed		
	Mean £ per week	sd	N*	Mean £ per week	sd	N*
Father's gross earnings	342	270	333	324	191	296
Father's net earnings	257	238	330	228	117	293
Partner's gross earnings	192	125	128	189	121	111
Partner's net earnings	141	80	120	136	77	107
Father's and partner's gross earnings	402	314	318	385	252	284
Father's and partner's net earnings	297	262	312	272	163	281
Benefits	56	47	270	59	47	246
Income from other sources	37	36	62	34	35	57
Total gross income	314	307	430	295	259	397
Total net income	241	247	424	219	170	394
Net disposable income (NDI)	228	244	411	205	163	382
NDI after child support	208	233	404	185	145	375
NDI after housing costs	183	224	365	165	137	344
NDI after child support and housing costs	163	216	357	146	120	336
Equivalent net income (HBAI scales)	298	368	424	264	214	394

* The numbers vary due to excluding cases where the data have not been provided.

Benefits

About half the fathers (52 per cent) were receiving some kind of social security benefit. Thirty per cent had children in their household and were therefore receiving Child Benefit, 2 per cent were also receiving One Parent Benefit, 3 per cent were also receiving Family Credit and 3 per cent Disabled Working Allowance. The most common out-of-work benefit received was Income Support – nearly a quarter of the fathers were dependent on Income Support, 2 per cent were receiving Unemployment Benefit and 6 per cent Invalidity Benefit. Table 4.8 on page 62 summarises the receipt of benefit.

Of those fathers in receipt of Income Support, only one father reported any earnings (£17 per week), and none of the partners of those on Income Support had any earnings.

Other income

After taking account of income from benefits, other income was calculated. Eleven per cent of the fathers had income from another source,

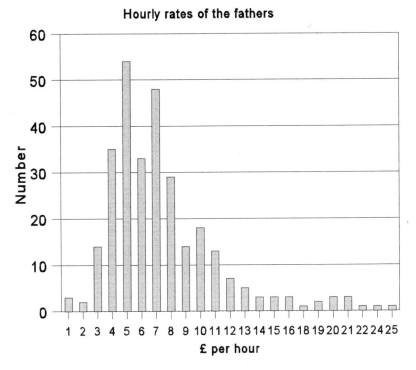

Figure 4.3 Frequency distribution of the hourly rates of pay for respondents

and these are summarised in Table 4.9 on page 63. It is interesting that twenty-five cases said that they were receiving payments from their new partner's last partner – that is 18 per cent of the fathers who were living with a partner with children from a previous partnership.

Total income

A variety of summary income variables was presented in Table 4.7. Net disposable income is net income after the deduction of travel-to-work costs and child-care expenses – 56 per cent of the fathers with earnings had travel costs, averaging £17 per week, and 58 per cent of their partners had travel-to-work costs, averaging £14 per week. Seven per cent of the households where either the fathers or their partners were working, had child-care costs averaging £35 per week. Also presented is net disposable income after housing costs. Average housing costs for tenants not on Income Support was £46 per week (sd = 37),

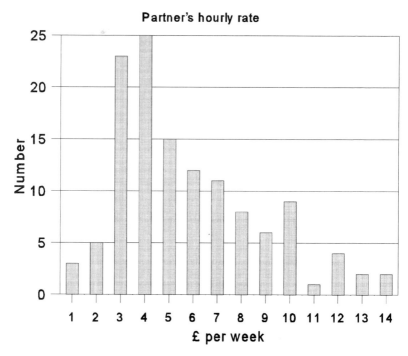

Figure 4.4 Distribution of the hourly rates of pay for partners

Table 4.8 Benefits received (including self-employed)

	Mean amount received £ per week	sd	% receiving each benefit	Number receiving
Income Support	63	29	22	127
Child Benefit	17	8	30	176
One Parent Benefit	6	0	2	13
Family Credit	48	30	3	16
Unemployment Benefit	61	18	2	13
Invalidity Benefit	70	33	6	37
Severe Disablement Allowance	34	11	1	3
Statutory Sick Pay	57	25	1	3
Statutory Maternity Pay	92	52	1	3
Invalid Care Allowance	49	25	1	3
Retirement Pension	103	57	1	4
Disabled Working Allowance	157	335	3	16
Other state benefits	50	24	3	17
Not receiving any benefits			48	271
All	57	47		565

Table 4.9 Other income (including self-employed)

	Mean £ per week	sd	% receiving	Number receiving
Payment from spouse's last partner	30	17	5	25
Allowance from YTS/employment Training/business start up	10		(2)	2
Private/occupational pension	62	49	2	12
Income from savings and investments	56	218	3	17
Rent from property	63	27	1	5
Other payments	65	61	2	9
All	37	36		62

Respondents may have other income from more than one source.
Figures in brackets are numbers.

for owner occupiers on Income Support it was £12 per week (sd = 21), and for owner occupiers not on Income Support it was £83 per week (sd = 44). In addition there is net disposable income after child support payments and housing costs. Taking only those who pay child support, then child support reduces net disposable income by an average of £30 per week. Taking only those who pay housing costs, then these costs reduce net disposable income by an average of £69 per week.

Finally, in order to compare the incomes of different types of household on a basis that takes account of their different needs, we use an equivalence scale. The equivalence scale[11] used in this analysis is the 'McClements Scale', which is the one employed by the Department of Social Security in its analysis of *Households Below Average Incomes*.

Table 4.10 compares the equivalent net income of the fathers according to their various characteristics. Fathers living in households with children only (who are therefore lone parents), households without an earner, and in particular fathers dependent on Income Support have the lowest equivalent net income. There is no difference in the net income of those fathers who have had and have not had contact with the Child Support Agency.

Additionally we see that the single, ex-cohabitants, those living alone, and particularly those dependent on Income Support, are more likely to be living below this threshold. Only 5 per cent of those not on Income Support, and none of those with two earners in the household, are living below the Income Support threshold.

Table 4.10 Equivalent net income (including self-employed)

	Mean £ per week	sd	% with equivalent net income below the Income Support threshold	N
Current marital status				
single	314	447	25	263
married	275	177	8	95
cohabiting	268	171	18	67
Marital status at split and now				
single/now married	146	97	(3)	5
single/now cohabiting	211	197	(1)	3
single/now single	214	151	29	38
married/now divorced	382	584	20	113
married/now separated	356	337	13	37
married/now cohabiting	292	170	10	50
married/now remarried	289	181	4	70
cohabiting/now separated	240	325	36	75
cohabiting/now cohabiting	192	156	39	13
cohabiting/now married	256	170	10	20
Household composition				
lives alone	346	390	25	161
lives with partner only	361	217	10	59
lives with partner/and child only	216	125	17	102
no partner, child only	145	84	16	19
lives with other/relatives no partner nor child	314	751	20	46
other	269	204	27	37
Earners				
no earners	108	63	58	134
one earner	386	474	3	189
two earners	385	274	—	101
on Income Support	92	38	67	103
not on Income Support	363	401	5	321
Contact with the CSA				
yes	299	456	20	185
no	299	283	20	237
All	298	368	20	424

Figures in brackets are numbers.

Distribution of income

Figure 4.5 provides a picture of net income and equivalent net income by decile group and shows that incomes are very widely dispersed – the HBAI equivalent income varies from a mean of £48 per week for those in the bottom decile to £881 per week for those in the top decile.

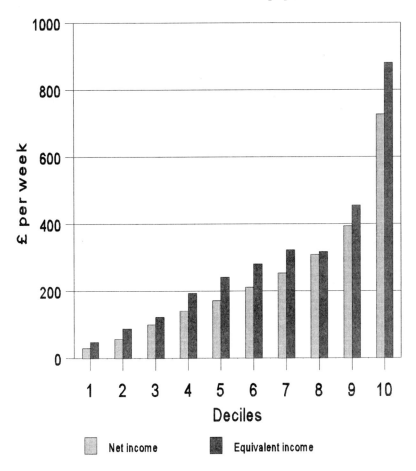

Figure 4.5 Income by deciles

Figure 4.6 shows how the components of net income vary over the income distribution – for the first three deciles income from benefits, particularly Income Support, is the most important contributor to net income. From the fourth decile fathers' earnings form the largest proportion of income. However, partners' earnings contribute over 20 per cent of the net income of the top three deciles.

Poverty rates

In order to evaluate the relative standard of living of the fathers, we take the mean equivalent net incomes of those in the study dependent

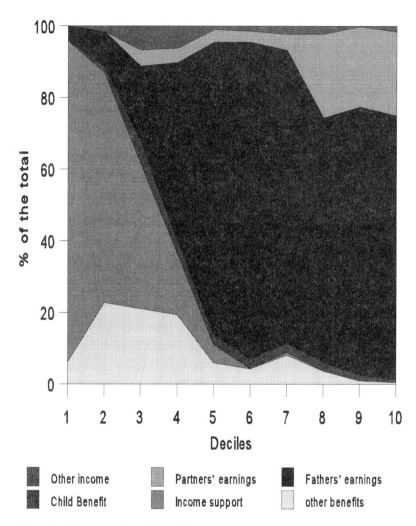

Figure 4.6 Sources of net disposable income

on Income Support as a poverty threshold, and then estimate the proportion of fathers' households with equivalent net income around this
threshold.[12] The results are summarised in Table 4.11. The poverty rate
varies with the threshold used, and with the income definition, but
20 per cent of the fathers have equivalent household net income below
this threshold and 37 per cent have equivalent net income, after child
support, housing costs, child-care and travel-to-work costs, below a
threshold only 20 per cent higher than the Income Support standard.

Table 4.11 Equivalent net income below various thresholds

	% with incomes less than 20% below the IS threshold	% with incomes below the IS threshold	% with incomes less than 20% above the IS threshold
Equivalent net income	7	20	27
Equivalent net income after deducting child support	9	22	29
Equivalent net income after housing costs	7	26	35
Equivalent net income after child support, housing costs, child-care and travel-to-work costs	14	27	37

Table 4.12 Access to assets

	Non-resident fathers %	All fathers in the Family Resources Survey 1994/95 %
One car	52	47
More than one car	19	42
Colour TV	92	99
Video player	85	95
Fridge/freezer	87	62
Freezer	28	49
Computer	29	43
Washing machine	86	98
Tumble dryer	46	70
Dishwasher	10	30
Phone	83	94
Number	587	6,288

Access to assets

One further indication of the living standards of non-resident fathers and their households can be obtained by examining the assets that they have access to. This is shown in Table 4.12 and a comparison is made with the assets that fathers in the Family Resources Survey have access to. It can be seen that a lower proportion of non-resident fathers have access to every one of the assets listed. They are more likely to have access to only one car rather than two or more and they are more likely to have a fridge/

freezer rather than a fridge and a separate freezer. In general these findings confirm that non-resident fathers are not as well off as fathers in general.

Feelings about financial situation

Those fathers who had a living-together relationship with their previous partners with whom they had children were asked to compare their financial situation when they were living together with now. The results are presented in Table 4.13, showing whether they felt better or worse off financially now. Forty-seven per cent said that they were worse off than when they were living together and these were more likely to describe their financial situation when they had lived together as comfortable. Just over a third of those who were better off now had been finding it difficult or very difficult when living with their last partner.

The fathers were also asked to describe their financial situation now. This is presented in Table 4.14. Nine per cent described themselves as very well off and 16 per cent as hard pressed. The latter group certainly

Table 4.13 Feelings about financial situation

Financial situation when living with last partner	Financial situation now			
	Worse off than when together %	Better off now %	Just the same %	All %
Living comfortably	47	16	11	27
Doing all right	25	15	33	23
Just about getting by	23	35	36	30
Finding it quite difficult	2	20	11	11
Finding it very difficult	4	15	8	9
All %	42	40	19	

Table 4.14 Current financial situation

	Equivalent net income £ per week	sd	% with equivalent net incomes below the IS threshold	% of the total
Very well off	406	238	2	9
Comfortably off	455	693	11	18
Managing all right	277	244	17	43
Not very well off	260	317	25	14
Hard pressed	155	127	44	16
All N = 432	298	368	20	100

had lower mean equivalent net incomes and 44 per cent of them were living below the Income Support threshold. Curiously, 11 per cent of the fathers describing themselves as comfortably off were also living below the IS threshold.

SUMMARY

In this chapter we have explored the employment and income of non-resident fathers. They are much less likely to be in employment and their employment status tends to be lower than fathers in general. Their partners are as likely to be in employment as the partners of resident fathers, but of course resident fathers are much more likely to have partners, and the partners of resident fathers tend to have higher-status jobs.

Non-resident fathers are on average likely to be low paid, dependent on social security benefits and, particularly after account is taken of unavoidable expenses such as travel to work, child support payments and child-care costs, living in poverty.

It has not been possible to use income to compare how much worse off the non-resident fathers were than fathers in general, because this survey was not a specialist survey of income, and it would be inappropriate to compare our results with those derived from a specialist survey such as the Family Expenditure Survey or the Family Resources Survey. However, the sources of the income of these fathers, particularly the high level of dependence on Income Support and other means-tested benefits, indicate that they are substantially worse off than resident fathers. Their hourly rate of pay is lower and they are also less likely to have access to a range of assets than fathers in general. This has implications for their standards of living, but particularly, as we shall see in Chapter 8, for their capacity to pay child support.

5   Housing

INTRODUCTION

If two parents have lived together before they separate, then there is inevitably a change in the housing circumstances of one or both of them. There is evidence that the housing consequences of relationship breakdown are one of the principal sources of stress experienced by lone mothers (Bradshaw and Millar, 1991; Bull, 1993), and these and other studies (Buck, 1994; Burrows, 1998; Holmans, 1990, 1995; McCarthy and Simpson, 1991; Sullivan, 1986; Symon, 1990) have depicted the tendency for lone mothers to move down the housing market – out of owner occupied and private rented dwellings, and into local authority or housing association dwellings. Separation is an important cause of rent and mortgage arrears (Boleat, 1985; Duncan and Kirby, 1983), repossessions (Ford, Kempson and Wilson, 1995) and homelessness (Ford, 1997; Greve and Currie, 1990). However, there is evidence (Holmans, 1990, 1995) that marital breakdown is more likely to occur among tenants, and studies of lone mothers have also shown that the vast majority of those already in social housing at the time of relationship breakdown, stayed in social housing, though not necessarily the same house. For married parents there is a tendency for the resident parent (almost invariably the mother) to take over the tenancy. For cohabiting parents, especially when the tenancy is in the name of the father, the position is more complicated, but local authority allocation policies would tend to favour the resident parent.

But what happens to non-resident fathers? There is some evidence that their status as non-resident means that their housing problems are even worse than those of lone mothers (Bull, 1993). If they had been a joint tenant of social housing, it is unlikely they will be a priority for rehousing in social housing. If they were owner occupiers, then the normal pattern on separation is either to split the equity, or to allocate more than half the equity and the house to the resident parent.

This is not just a private matter. The demand for extra dwellings generated by relationship breakdown and parents not living together in the same dwelling is enormous. Holmans (1990) estimated that dwellings for an extra 700,000 independent households were required at any one time, as a result of the breakdown of marriages, let alone the extra households required as a result of cohabitation breakdown and partners deciding not to live with the other parent of their children. As Bradshaw and Millar (1991) asserted:

> Together relationship breakdown and repartnering contribute a considerable proportion of the dynamism in the housing market and a substantial contribution to administrative burdens on housing authorities, housing associations, building societies, solicitors, the courts, advice agencies and social workers.
>
> (Bradshaw and Millar, 1991: 88)

Although some evidence on the housing circumstances of non-resident fathers has emerged from studies of lone mothers (Bradshaw and Millar, 1991), it has been partial because lone mothers do not always know what the circumstances of the father of their child are. Studies of divorcing couples have looked at what happens to housing (Eekelaar and Maclean, 1986; Maclean, 1987; Southwell, 1985; Sullivan, 1986), but they have tended to concentrate on the outcomes for the resident parent. The Bull and Stone (1989) study has some information on non-resident fathers from their qualitative interviews. So this study is the first opportunity to observe the housing consequences of all types of non-resident father.

Present tenure

The present tenure position of the non-resident fathers is summarised in Table 5.1, by their marital status at the time of their separation/child birth. Compared with all fathers there is a much lower proportion of non-resident fathers living in owner occupied dwellings, and a much higher proportion living with family and friends, and in all types of rented accommodation. However, 45 per cent of the non-resident fathers were living in owner occupied accommodation, which is a higher proportion than lone mothers. Bradshaw and Millar (1991) found that only 28 per cent of lone parents were owner occupiers. Non-resident fathers are also more likely to be living in private rented accommodation, and less likely to be local authority tenants than lone parents. Remarkably, a third of single non-resident fathers were living with family or friends. The ex-married were more likely to be owner occupiers than the single

Table 5.1 Present tenure of non-resident fathers, by marital status at the time of separation/child birth

	Single	Cohabiting	Married	Total	Tenure of fathers in the FRS
	%	%	%	%	%
Living with family/friends	32	16	8	12	2
Owned outright	(1)	5	5	4	7
Owned with mortgage	25	27	48	41	70
Local authority rented	21	25	21	22	14
Housing association rented	9	4	6	6	2
Private rented	12	22	10	13	5
Rent free	0	(1)	2	1	1
Bed and breakfast	0	0	(3)	(3)	0
Total	100	100	100	100	100
Base	(57)	(138)	(394)	(589)	(6,558)

Figures in brackets are numbers.

Table 5.2 Present tenure of non-resident fathers, by living arrangement

	Living alone	With partner only	With partner + child only	With child only	With parents only	Other	Total
	%	%	%	%	%	%	%
Living with family/friends					89	36	11
Owned outright	6	7	3		7	(1)	5
Owned with mortgage	45	62	47	22	(1)	19	41
Local authority rented	25	6	34	48	(1)	9	22
Housing association rented	6	7	7	17		(1)	6
Privately rented	16	11	8	(3)		30	13
Rent free with job	2	(3)	(1)				1
Bed and breakfast	(2)					(1)	(3)
Total	100	100	100	100	100	100	100
Number	215	93	151	23	54	53	589

Figures in brackets are numbers.

or ex-cohabiting, and the ex-cohabiting were more likely to be private tenants. There was little difference in the proportion of each marital status group living in local authority rented accommodation.

Table 5.2 shows that the majority of those living with family or friends were in fact living with their parents – they had 'gone back home' (or conceivably had never left). Those who had (re)partnered, but were without a new child, were most likely to be owners, and those who were living with a child only were much more likely to be social tenants (local authority or housing association). Nevertheless, about a third of non-resident fathers, living alone, were living in social housing.

Movements in tenure

Table 5.3 compares the accommodation of the parents before the split, with where they are living now (forty-six fathers did not know what type of accommodation their ex-partner occupied). For the fathers there was a net movement out of owner occupied and local authority dwellings, and a net movement into private rented and living with family and friends. For the former partners there was a movement out of owner occupied dwellings and into local authority, housing association and privately rented dwellings. However, 17 per cent of the fathers said they had been rehoused by a local authority or housing association. Most of these (56 per cent) were in social housing before the split but a quarter were owners. Nearly all of those rehoused (89 per cent) were still living in social housing.

Table 5.4 provides a more detailed breakdown of the movements between tenures. Half of those who had been living with family and friends before the split continued to live with them, but just over a quarter moved into owner occupied housing. Only a quarter of those

Table 5.3 Non-resident fathers' and their ex-partners' tenure before the split and now (excludes those who do not know their ex-partners' tenure)

	Before the split %	Father now %	Ex-partner now %
Family and friends	6	12	6
Owned outright	6	5	4
Owned with mortgage	46	41	34
Local authority rented	26	21	34
Housing association rented	6	6	8
Private rented	7	13	11
Rent free	1	1	2
Bed and breakfast/other	(5)	(3)	(2)
Base	(544)	(543)	(544)

Figures in brackets are numbers.

Table 5.4 Type of accommodation before becoming a non-resident father compared with type of accommodation now

Accommodation now	Accommodation before split									
	With friends/family %	Owned outright %	Owned with mortgage %	Local authority rented %	Housing association rented %	Private rented %	Rent free %	Bed and breakfast %	Hostel/don't know %	Total %
With friends/family	51	3	5	12	18	15				11
Owned outright		25	6	2			(3)			5
Owned with mortgage	27	41	64	19	27	21	(3)		(2)	42
Local authority rented	16	16	11	47	18	15			(1)	22
Housing association rented	(1)	(1)	4	4	24	15	(2)			6
Private rented	(1)	(3)	10	15	(4)	31		(1)	(1)	13
Rent free		(1)	(1)	(2)	(1)		(3)			1
Bed and breakfast			(1)			(2)				(3)
Total number	37	32	259	155	34	48	11	1	4	581
Total %	6	6	45	27	6	8	2	(1)	1	100

Figures in brackets are numbers.

Table 5.5 Proportions of ex-partners and respondents remaining in the accommodation they occupied before the split, by tenure (those with a living-together relationship only)

	Ex-partner %	Respondent %	Neither %	N
Living with family/friends	13	25	63	8
Owned outright	24	29	48	21
Owned with mortgage	38	20	42	230
Local authority rented	44	12	45	131
Rented from housing association	46	9	46	33
Rented from private landlord	20	(2)	74	35
Rent free, bed and breakfast/don't know	(1)	(1)	(7)	8
Total	37	16	47	467

Figures in brackets are numbers.

who owned outright continued to own outright, but most of the rest became owners with a mortgage. Just less than two-thirds of owners with a mortgage remained owners with a mortgage, but 15 per cent found their way into social housing. Less than half the local authority tenants, and less than a quarter of housing association tenants, retained their tenancies, but the most common outcome for them was a move into owner occupation, although significant proportions also moved in with friends and relatives or into the private rented sector. A third of those who had been private renters before the split stayed private renters, and the most common other outcome was to move into owner occupation. So the general picture is rather mixed – a good deal of evidence of change, but not necessarily always change that can be described as down-market.

So far we have looked at the types of accommodation occupied now, compared with the types occupied before the split. This tells us something about the proportions of non-resident fathers who shifted tenure, but it does not tell us much about moves – a father staying in the same tenure does not necessarily imply that he stayed in the same dwelling or area. In Table 5.5 we restrict the analysis to those non-resident fathers who had had a living-together relationship (married or cohabiting) before they split with their partners. It shows that the mothers were much more likely to retain the accommodation than fathers – 37 per cent compared with 16 per cent – and that they were particularly more likely to retain the dwelling if they were living in social housing. Only fathers living with family or friends, and those who were outright owners, were more likely than the mothers to retain their accommodation. However, the picture confirms the results of previous studies that relationship breakdown results in major disruption in housing circumstances. In nearly half of the living-together relationships, neither they nor their partner were still living in the family accommodation after the split.

Number of moves

Also, a father shifting tenure could have moved a number of times. At the time of the interview only 15 per cent had lived in one place since becoming a non-resident father, and another third (34 per cent) had lived in two places. In contrast, 14 per cent of fathers had moved at least five times, and one father had moved twenty-one times. The number of moves of course is associated with the length of non-resident father-hood. Of those fathers who had been non-resident for less than two years, 62 per cent had lived in only one place, whereas of those who had been non-resident fathers for 10 years or more, only 10 per cent had lived in one place.

Arrears

Of those with experience of renting since the split, 46 per cent of those who had been in local authority housing, 62 per cent of those in housing association dwellings and 38 per cent of those in private land-lord dwellings had experienced arrears in their rent of at least a month (not shown). Over a third (35 per cent) of the fathers who had lived as owner occupiers had been in mortgage arrears of at least a month. Arrears with local rates/community charge/council tax were also common – 29 per cent of the fathers had been in council tax arrears since the split; and it was more common among those who had been in social housing at some time – 55 per cent of housing association tenants and 41 per cent of council tenants had been in arrears. About a fifth of the fathers (22 per cent) had been in mortgage arrears. However, threats of eviction were much less common – 7 per cent of owners had been threatened with repossession and 20 per cent of local authority tenants, 18 per cent of housing association tenants, and 4 per cent of private tenants had been threatened with eviction. But only eight fathers in the study had actually experienced eviction/repossession, most of whom appear to have been evicted from private rented accommodation.

Satisfaction with housing

Despite the volatility of the housing experiences of the non-resident fathers following their relationship breakdown, there was a remarkable

Table 5.6 Satisfaction with present accommodation, by tenure

| | *Very satisfied or fairly satisfied* | *Much better or better than accommodation when the child was born* | *Worse or much worse than the accommodation when the child was born* |
	%	%	%
Living with family/friends	76	32	20
Owned outright	88	34	15
Owned with mortgage	88	43	17
Local authority rented	68	37	32
Housing association rented	75	31	23
Private rented	55	37	49
Rent free	88	37	(1)
Bed and breakfast	(2)	0	(2)
All %	77	38	25
Base	588	575	575

Figures in brackets are numbers.

level of satisfaction with their current accommodation. It can be seen in Table 5.6 that 77 per cent of the non-resident fathers were very satisfied or fairly satisfied. Levels of satisfaction were highest among owner occupiers, and lowest among private renters. Over a third (38 per cent) also felt that their accommodation was much better or better than they had been living in when the child was born or the split occurred, and only a quarter felt that it was worse or much worse. Again, private renters were the only tenure group to have a larger proportion thinking that their accommodation was worse than those thinking it was better. These levels of satisfaction with housing are almost identical to those found among lone parents by Bradshaw and Millar (1991).

Table 5.7 shows how satisfaction varied by change in tenure. Those who remained owner occupiers and those who moved from renting to owning were most likely to be satisfied (apart from those who moved from renting to other arrangements), and those who remained renters, or who moved from owning to renting, were most likely to be dissatisfied. Over half of the very dissatisfied group were those who had remained renters (not shown). Of those who moved from owning to renting, 63 per cent of them said it was worse or much worse than their previous accommodation, compared with 25 per cent overall. However, there were some, who had remained owners or who had become owners, who were also dissatisfied, and 20 per cent of those who remained owners said that their housing was worse or much worse than

Table 5.7 Satisfaction with accommodation, by change in housing tenure

	Owner to owner %	Renter to owner %	Owner to renter %	Renter to renter %	Owner to other %	Renter to other %	Other %	All %
Very satisfied	48	48	25	32	40	51	43	40
Fairly satisfied	41	39	41	37	(5)	14	43	37
Neither satisfied nor dissatisfied	6		9	8		14	2	7
Fairly dissatisfied	4	6	12	11	(2)	17	6	8
Very dissatisfied	2	4	12	15	(2)	3	6	8
Number	200	52	75	157	15	35	51	585
%	37	8	13	27	3	6	15	100

before the split. This suggests that for some non-resident fathers it was not necessarily a blessing to become owner occupiers, perhaps because of the lack of alternative choices or the relative costs of the different tenures.

Taking only those who had experienced a living-together relationship with their partners (married or cohabiting), then just over a third of the sample (38 per cent) lived in owner occupier accommodation before they split. We asked them to describe how the equity in the dwelling had been split – 29 per cent said that their partner had taken the whole property value, and only 9 per cent said that they had taken the whole value. In the other cases the value was shared and 12 per cent had not yet settled the issue. It is not surprising that the formerly married were most likely to be the ones where the partner took the whole property, and the formerly cohabiting were more likely to have taken the whole property value themselves (not shown).

SUMMARY

The housing consequences of relationship breakdown are profound. Over 80 per cent of those fathers who had been living with their partners before the split had had to move, and many had experienced multiple moves, drifting between different types of accommodation. A remarkably high proportion (56 per cent) had had to rely at some point on family and friends, and also a period in private rented accommodation was very common. Non-resident fathers were much less likely than lone parents to find a refuge in social housing. However, as with lone parents, there is clear evidence of a drift down-market, with about half the proportion of non-resident fathers living as owner occupiers compared with fathers in general.

Nevertheless, despite rent and mortgage arrears being common, evictions and repossession threatened, and a few actual evictions, more non-resident fathers than their partners were owner occupiers at the time of the interview, and a quarter had obtained access to social housing. Further, the levels of satisfaction with their current housing were high – only 17 per cent were not satisfied with their housing (exactly the same proportion found among lone parents by Bradshaw and Millar, 1991), and only a quarter felt that their accommodation now was worse than that they had occupied before becoming a non-resident father.

6 Contact between non-resident fathers and their children

INTRODUCTION

One of the most important issues to be investigated in this study was the extent and quality of the contact between the non-resident fathers and their children. Certain barriers have to be overcome by the non-resident father if he is to maintain contact with his children – both practical and emotional – and they have to be surmounted in order for the non-resident father to be able to function cooperatively as a parent with his ex-partner. In this chapter we draw on the results of the sample survey and in the next chapter we employ material from the qualitative study that focused on contact to explore the issue further.

Simpson *et al.* (1995), using data collected before the instigation of the Child Support Act in 1993, found that the strongest indicators of contact were the father's occupational status and level of income. The higher the employment status, the more the fathers were likely to have regular contact with their children. They found that 74 per cent of unemployed fathers had little or no contact with their children. The higher the income, the more likely it was for children to have overnight stays. They found no apparent link between maintenance payments and quantity and type of contact. Of the fathers who had little or no contact, 74 per cent were angry about this and wanted to change contact arrangements. However, the no-contact fathers, who had given up the battle over contact, adjusted most easily to divorce and repartnered more readily. This option of the 'clean break' and dropping out of parental responsibility is no longer viable since the Child Support Act 1991.

However, evidence provided by Seltzer (1991) and Seltzer, Schaeffer and Charng (1989) in North America suggested that maintenance and contact are positively correlated, and that separated fathers combine their responsibilities on three parameters: social contact, financial involvement and participation in parental decision making.

Table 6.1 How often did the non-resident father see his children?

	%
At least once a week	47
At least once a fortnight	14
At least once a month	7
Once or twice a year	10
1–3 years	8
More than three years	10
Not at all	3
Base number	620

Level of contact

A major grievance of fathers in this sample, certainly more important than concerns over child support, was the difficulties that they had seeing their children. Nevertheless contact with their non-resident children was rather higher than expected (Table 6.1). Only 21 per cent of our sample had not seen their children in the last year and 47 per cent saw their child at least every week.

This is evidence of a much higher level of contact than that derived from studies of lone parents. For example, Bradshaw and Millar (1991) found that lone parents said that 57 per cent of all non-resident parents had contact currently with their children. They also found that the proportion with contact tended to decline with the length of lone parenthood – for example, of those who had been lone parents for over two years and less than three years 40 per cent of non-resident parents had no contact. These findings have been much quoted in discussions about the consequences of family breakdown. The findings of this study, that only 3 per cent had no contact at all, suggest that there might be something very wrong with the reliability of the results in this study or Bradshaw and Millar's or both. We therefore need to start by attempting to reconcile these findings.

First, it is important to remember that the samples are not matched. Bradshaw and Millar's study contained both male and female lone parents, and the proportion having contact was lower among the non-resident fathers (56 per cent) than among the non-resident mothers (72 per cent). Further, in this study, the ex-partners of non-resident fathers are not necessarily lone mothers – thus the sample of fathers is not matched by a sample of lone mothers. We found that 86 per cent of the non-resident fathers knew the present circumstances of their ex-partner, and in 57 per cent of these cases the ex-partner had repartnered and was no longer a lone mother. So we would expect to find some differences in the contact levels of the fathers in this study and of the fathers to the children of lone mothers in the Bradshaw and Millar (1991) study.

Second, the questions about contact were not identical in the two surveys. In Bradshaw and Millar (1991) respondents were asked 'Does your last partner with whom you had children ever see the children that live with you? If no, when did your former (last) partner last see the children? If yes, about how often does your former partner see the children?' In this study the fathers were asked 'When did you last see your children from this relationship?' If the answer is over one year they are then asked 'Why is it that you have not seen your children for over a year?' If the answer is less than one year, then there are questions about distance and shared care and then 'How often do you see the children?' In the Bradshaw and Millar (1991) study some lone parents said that the fathers did not see their child, but when asked when the father last saw their child, the lone mothers said that it was within the last six months. Similarly in this study there were nine fathers who said that they last saw their children within the last four weeks, who normally see the children only once a year or less. Also there were six fathers who said that they normally see their children once week but had last seen them more than four weeks ago. These seemingly contradictory statements in both the surveys are in fact possible. They could be the result of a fairly short episode of non-resident fatherhood/lone parenthood, or because the contact arrangements have changed since the last contact, or because the last contact just happened to be fairly recent or because the father was away.

More profoundly, the emphasis on *seeing* the child in the questions about contact may be, with hindsight, too imprecise a definition of contact, failing to pick up the essence of a relationship between the fathers and their children. As we shall see later, *seeing* encompasses the range between sighting your child walking to school, or going on a week's holiday once a year, to totally shared care. Seeing did not perhaps pick up on alternative ways of maintaining a fairly close, and perhaps valued relationship, between the fathers and their children, including regular phoning, correspondence and even e-mail.

Nevertheless, in an attempt to reconcile the differences between the two surveys, we decided to reanalyse the Bradshaw and Millar (1991) survey in order to produce estimates of contact, just for the fathers of the children of lone mothers, and to match it to the classification of contact used in this present study. The results are summarised in Table 6.2. Even after adjusting both data sets so that they match, there are considerable differences in the distributions. In particular, the

Table 6.2 Comparisons of contact reported by lone mothers and
non-resident fathers

	Lone mothers reporting their child seeing their father (Bradshaw and Millar 1991) %	Non-resident fathers reporting seeing their child %
At least once a week	27	47
At least once a fortnight	7	14
At least once a month	7	7
At least once a year	24	10
1–3 years	10	8
More than three years ago	10	10
Never	11	3
Don't know	4	1
Number	1,360	626

proportion of fathers saying that they see their children at least weekly is nearly twice that reported by lone mothers, and the proportion of fathers saying that they never see their child is less than a third that reported by lone mothers.

However, contact levels vary considerably by marital status. The proportion of children *not* seeing their fathers in the last month was 51 per cent among the ex-married, 54 per cent among the ex-cohabiting and 75 per cent among the single lone mothers in the Bradshaw and Millar (1991) study, and single never married lone mothers constitute 39 per cent of the lone mothers sample compared with only 10 per cent of single never married fathers in this study. So in Table 6.3 we compare contact levels, having controlled for the marital status of the mothers and fathers. This reduces the difference to some extent, but there is still a substantial difference in the proportion not seeing their children at least monthly, and it is consistently lower for each marital status group in this study of non-resident fathers.

There is also an association between contact and the length of lone parenthood: in the lone mother sample two-thirds of the children of lone mothers who had been separated for more than three years had not seen their fathers for more than a month compared with just under a half of those who had been separated for less than a year. In the fathers sample, of those separated from their children for over three years 38 per cent had not seen their child in the last month compared with only 16 per cent of those who had been non-resident fathers for less than a year. So after controlling for length of lone motherhood/non-resident fathering there is still a fairly substantial difference between

Table 6.3 Proportion of fathers not having contact with their children in the last month, by marital status

Marital status	Lone mothers in Bradshaw and Millar (1991) %	Non-resident fathers %
Ex–single	75	49
Ex–married	51	28
Ex–cohabiting	54	38
Length of lone motherhood/non-resident fatherhood		
less than a year	46	16
1–3 years	55	19
more than three years	67	38
Separated more than three years		
ex–single	77	59
ex–married	60	33
ex–cohabiting	64	42
All	61	32
Number	1,360	620

the surveys. In fact the fathers in our sample had been separated from the mothers of their children for rather longer than the sample of lone mothers had been separated from the fathers of their children. Thus one might have expected our sample of fathers to be less, not more, likely to be in contact with their children. The differences are not resolved when marital status and length of separation are simultaneously controlled for. For example, comparing the ex-married and those who have been separated for at least three years in each sample, we find that 60 per cent have not seen their father in the last month in Bradshaw and Millar (1991) compared with 33 per cent in this present study.

There are three possible explanations for the differences observed. First, the fact that they are not matched samples, as has been explained above. Then there is the possibility that this sample was biased in favour of men with contact – those without contact could well have been men reluctant to acknowledge that they were the father of a child in another household at the screening survey. Finally, perhaps lone mothers and non-resident fathers perceive and report contact differently – lone mothers may not welcome, and be reluctant to acknowledge, the continuing involvement of a non-resident father. Or they may feel that the nature of that contact is too trivial to recognise. In contrast, the fathers may want to assert their parental role, and perhaps claim greater involvement than in reality they have. To the caring parent, contact may mean a share of caring. But to the non-resident parent it may be merely a brief (fatherly) social interaction.

We have sought to find a framework for understanding the barriers to contact, and have speculated on certain factors that would influence contact. Some of these are factors that have been found by researchers in North America and Australia – for example Selzter (1991) in the US suggests that maintenance and contact are positively correlated, and Sutton (1996) in Australia has shown that after income there are two factors that are important – the relationship with the ex-partner and the feeling of loss of control.

Table 6.4 presents an analysis of the factors that we speculated would

Table 6.4 Factors influencing regular contact with a child

Variable	Bivariate	Simultaneous	Best-fitting
Quintiles			
1	1.00	1.00	
2	0.96	2.12	
3	1.93★	2.03	
4	1.57	1.41	
5	2.73★★	3.01	
not known	1.12	2.05	
Marital status now			
single	1.00	1.00	
married	0.39★★★	0.79	
cohabiting	0.63★	0.93	
Family composition			
children	1.00	1.00	1.00
no children	2.09★★	1.92	2.16★
living alone	2.82★★★	2.42	2.80★★
Marital status at child's birth			
cohabiting	1.00	1.00	
married	1.60★	2.69★★	
single	0.94	1.43	
Age first became father			
under 20	1.00	1.00	
20–24	2.03★	0.50	
25–30	3.06★★★	0.89	
31+	3.15★★★	0.85	
Employment status			
employed	1.00	1.00	1.00
self-employed	0.80	0.46	0.54
inactive	0.54★★	0.64	0.49★
Age of youngest child			
0–4	1.00	1.00	
5–10	0.60★	0.76	
11–18	0.46★★	0.44	

Table 6.4 (cont'd)

Variable	Bivariate	Simultaneous	Best-fitting
Sex of children			
only boys	1.00	1.00	
only girls	1.43	1.30	
girls and boys	1.76★	2.28★	
Number of children			
one	1.00	1.00	
two	1.18	0.28★★★	
three or more	1.74	0.21★	
Time to travel to child			
under 10 mins	1.00	1.00	1.00
10 mins–half hour	0.61	0.76	0.78
half an hour–1 hour	0.43	0.48	0.47★
1–2 hours	0.16★★★	0.17★★	0.19★★★
2 hours+	0.04★★★	0.03★★★	0.04★★★
Length of non-resident parenthood			
1–2 years	1.00	1.00	
3–5 years	0.47★	1.02	
6–9 years	0.26★★★	0.60	
10+ years	0.16★★★	0.68	
How often see family			
weekly	1.00	1.00	
once a month	1.89	0.49	
three monthly to yearly	0.49★★	0.89	
less often or never	0.49★★	0.39★	

★$p < 0.05$; ★★$p < 0.01$; ★★★$p < 0.001$.

influence contact. The bivariate analysis takes each variable in turn and shows how the proportion having regular contact (defined as at least monthly) varies – thus, for example, fathers living alone are 2.8 times more likely to have regular contact than a father living in a household with children, or fathers who have (re)married are two-thirds less likely to see children from their previous partnerships. In addition, fathers who were older when they first became fathers, employed fathers, fathers with younger children, fathers who live close to the child, who pay maintenance, and who have an amicable relationship with their ex-partner, are much more likely to have regular contact with their absent child.

However, a number of these factors interact, and so the next two columns present the results of logistic regression. In the best-fitting model the time taken to visit, employment status, and the new family composition, are the ones to emerge. Fathers are much more likely to have contact with their non-resident children if they live alone or just with a partner, if they are in employment, and if they live within half an hour's journey time of the child. Income and length of time as a non-resident father, while significant factors affecting contact in the bivariate analysis, do not emerge as significant after controlling for the other factors. Also, contact with the fathers' own family did not appear to be as important as had been expected from the qualitative analysis (see Chapter 7), when all other things were held constant.

Two factors were left out of the analysis above despite the fact that they were very closely associated with contact. These are the relationship between the non-resident parent and their ex-partner and whether maintenance is paid. They were left out of the model on the grounds that they are not unrelated to contact with the child – they may be the result as well as the cause of contact. Nevertheless, the relationship with the mother is, not surprisingly, a crucial determinant of regularity of contact with the child.

Relationship with the mother

Seventy-one per cent of the fathers said that they still had some contact with the mothers of their children. About half of those with contact (49 per cent) described their relationship with their former partner as amicable, and another quarter as amicable but distant. Only 18 per cent described the relationship as distant and hostile, hostile or non-existent. A logistic regression was undertaken to explore the factors affecting the nature of the relationship with the former partner. In Table 6.5 it can be seen that in the best-fitting model, having controlled for all the other variables, only two variables emerge as significant (at the 99 per cent level) – the time it takes to visit the child and the father's present family circumstances – fathers who live over an hour away and who are now living in households with children have less amicable relations with their former partner than those who live alone or with a new partner without children. It appears from this that new children and new step-children may result in a deterioration in relationships with former partners, and compete for time and attention with the absent children.

Of those fathers with some contact with their former partners, 64 per cent communicated with them at least once a week, and the more amicable the relationship, the more regular the communication. Nevertheless 46 per cent of those fathers with a hostile relationship also communicated at least once a week. As would be expected, there was also a close association between communication with the former partner and seeing the absent child – 91 per cent of the fathers who saw their child every week, communicated with their former partner at least once a fortnight (not shown). However, there were some cases where

Table 6.5 Relationship with the mother

Variable	Bivariate	Simultaneous	Best-fitting
Quintile			
1	1.00	1.00	
2	0.83	0.78	
3	1.05	0.97	
4	1.17	1.06	
5	1.77	1.22	
not known	1.60	2.61	
Time lived with child			
never lived together/separated			
before child born	1.00	1.00	
separated within 1 year	0.83★★★	0.80	
1–3 years	0.82★★★	0.81	
3–6 years	1.44★★★	0.87	
over 6 years	1.90	1.00	
Marital status at child's birth			
cohabiting	1.00	1.00	1.00
married	1.60	1.82	1.77★
single	1.46★★★	2.06	2.83★
Age when first became father			
under 20	1.00	1.00	
20–24	1.75	1.06	
25–30	2.06	1.00	
31+	1.91	0.91	
Employment status			
employed	1.00	1.00	
self-employed	0.92★★★	0.58	
inactive	0.73	0.98	
Age of youngest child			
0–4	1.00	1.00	
5–10	0.87★★★	0.83	
11–18	1.23★★★	1.01	
Length of absent fatherhood			
1–2 years	1.00	1.00	
3–5 years	0.79★★★	1.07	
6–9 years	0.80★★★	1.68	
10+ years	0.61★	1.63	
How often sees relatives			
once a week	1.00	1.00	
at least once a month	0.86	0.99	
three months to yearly	0.89	1.50	
less often/never	0.89	1.03	
Number of children			
one	1.00	1.00	
two	0.99★★★	0.58	
three or more	1.20★★★	0.65	
Family			
with children	1.00	1.00	1.00
no children	1.57★	1.30	1.60
lives alone	2.26★★★	1.52	1.96★★

Table 6.5 *(cont'd)*

Variable	Bivariate	Simultaneous	Best-fitting
Sex of children			
only boys	1.00	1.00	
only girls	1.02	0.92	
boys and girls	1.07	1.05	
Journey time to see child			
<10 mins	1.00	1.00	1.00
10 mins–half an hour	0.59*	0.62	0.64
half an hour–1 hour	0.73	1.00	0.93
1–2 hours	0.28***	0.25***	0.31***
2 hours+	0.42**	0.35**	0.44**
Marital status			
single	1.00	1.00	
married	0.48	0.42	
cohabiting	0.77***	0.82	

*p < 0.05; **p < 0.01; ***p < 0.001.

the father saw his child every week, but communication with the mother was much less regular – thus eleven fathers who saw their child at least once a fortnight said that they communicated with their former partner once or twice a year or less. One wonders at the difficulty of organising the contact with the child without communication with the resident parent. There were very few cases where communication with partners was regular but the father did not see the child – in only one case was there communication with the mother at least weekly and no contact whatsoever with the child.

Similar to what we have seen in relation to contact with the children, there was evidence that geographical distance between the fathers and their former partners was a factor in determining the relationship between the parents. These results are summarised in Table 6.6. Those fathers who described their relationship as distant or distant but hostile or non-existent lived further away from their partners than those who described the relationship as amicable. However, those who described their relationship as merely hostile were on average nearer their partners than those with amicable relationships. This may suggest that distance in relationships is associated with spatial distance, rather than necessarily an emotional distance, which was meant by the question. There was a somewhat clearer relationship between the regularity of communication and distance. Thus those fathers who communicated with their former partner at least weekly lived on average 26 miles away, whereas those who communicated only once or twice a year lived on average 101 miles away.

Table 6.6 Relationship and communication with former partner, by distance from former partner

Relationship with former partner	Distance from former partner (miles)	sd	All % n = 613	How often do you communicate	Distance from former partner	sd	All % n = 441
Amicable	34	92	36	At least once a week	26	78	64
Amicable but distant	32	79	19	At least once a fortnight	23	56	11
Distant	60	115	9	At least once a month	56	103	11
Distant but hostile	74	134	9	At least every three months	118	182	6
Hostile	19	44	11	Once or twice a year	101	137	7
No relationship	67	120	16	Less often	76	102	(2)
				Not at all	13	24	(6)
All	42	98	100	All	39	96	100

Figures in brackets are numbers.

Table 6.7 Reasons given for not seeing the child

	% of cases	% of responses
Mother obstructs contact	53	47
Don't know where child is	12	11
Child does not want to see father	6	5
Court order prevents it	5	5
Don't want to see child	5	4
Never wanted child	2	2
Other	29	26
Number	101	112

Reasons for not seeing the child

Those fathers who had not seen their child for over a year – 17 per cent of the total – were asked their reasons for not seeing him or her (Table 6.7). The most common reason, given by over half the fathers, was that the mother obstructed access. In addition there were twelve fathers who did not know where their child was, six cases where the child did not want to see the father, five where the father did not want to see the child, and two who said that they never wanted the child. Only five fathers said that a court order prevented them seeing the child.

Shared care

There were thirty fathers in the sample (4.8 per cent of the total) who had an arrangement that could be described as shared care.[13] The most common arrangement was for the child to spend half the week with the father and half the week with the mother (ten fathers). In seven cases the child spent weekends with the father and the week with the mother. In one case the child spent alternate weeks with the mother and the father and the rest (thirteen cases) had some other arrangement. Although, given the small numbers involved, the differences are not statistically significant, those children who spent roughly equal periods of time with each of their parents tended to be younger, girls and only children, and the father was less likely to be living with a new partner – only 13 per cent (four) of the shared care group had a new partner compared with 40 per cent of those where the child spent much more time with the mother. Those with shared care were much more likely to feel that the amount they saw their children was 'about right' (72 per cent compared with only 45 per cent of those who did not share care). They were also much more likely to feel they had control over the amount of contact with their child (78 per cent compared with 54 per cent among those who did not share care).

Frequency of seeing the child

In response to the question 'When did you last see your child living in another household?' we were given the responses summarised in Table 6.8.

Table 6.8 Frequency of seeing child

	%	N
Today	12.3	77
This week	29.6	185
Last week	14.9	93
Within last two weeks	8.3	52
Within last month	5.2	33
Within last six months	8.0	50
Six months to one year ago	3.9	24
Between one and three years ago	5.6	35
More than three years ago	10.2	64
Never	0.9	5
Don't know/no response	1.1	7
All	100	625

Table 6.9 Frequency of seeing child, by satisfaction with contact

	% saying that contact with children about right	% feeling in control of the amount of contact	All %	N
At least once a week	66	64	57	255
At least once a fortnight	22	20	19	86
At least once a month	8	8	9	41
At least once every three months	3	5	8	37
Once or twice a year	(3)	3	6	28
%	47	56	100	446

We then excluded those with shared care and those with no contact in the last year, and analysed the frequency of contact with the child. It can be seen in Table 6.9 that over half (57 per cent) of fathers saw their child at least once a week and 76 per cent saw their child at least every two weeks. The fathers who saw their child most often were likely to be the ones who said that they thought that the frequency of contact was about right – only two fathers thought that they saw their child too often (both once a week). The rest – over half the fathers – said they did not see their child often enough, despite the fact that half of these saw the child at least once a week. About half the fathers (56 per cent) felt that they had control over the amount of contact with their child, and they were also the ones who were most likely to see their child most.

As we have already discussed, 'seeing a child' can mean a variety of different things. Those fathers who visited their child, or where the child visited them, were asked to describe how long they usually spend with the child. The results are summarised in Table 6.10, analysed by the frequency of visits. The most common pattern, experienced by over a third of the fathers/children, is for the father/child to stay up to two nights. But half of the visits do not involve overnight stays, and 7 per cent are brief – less than two hours. Even some irregular visits are relatively brief – thus 15 per cent of those who see their child only once a month see her/him for less than two hours. However, in general the more infrequent contacts tended to involve longer stays – thus, of those who see their child only every three months nearly half (49 per cent) stay over two nights.

Some fathers spend a longer time with their children during the school holidays than they normally do – about 55 per cent said that they did this, including 38 per cent of those who only spent under two hours with their children on normal visits. However, the fathers who

Table 6.10 Length of visits, by the frequency of the visits

	Under 2 hours %	*2–6 hours* %	*Up to a day, not overnight* %	*Up to two nights* %	*Over two nights* %	*N*
At least once a week	6	25	23	40	7	254
Once every two weeks	7	13	18	47	15	83
Once a month	15	20	17	27	22	41
Once every three months	(2)	14	20	11	49	35
Once–twice a year	10	35	20	20	15	20
All	7	22	21	37	14	433

Figures in brackets are numbers.

normally had their children to stay overnight were also those who were most likely to spend longer with them in the holidays.

Not seeing a child between visits does not necessarily imply that there is no contact between the father and the child. It can be seen in Table 6.11 that only 23 per cent of the fathers had no contact by telephone, letter or card with their child between visits (the age of the child is clearly a factor in this). It was also found (though not shown in Table 6.11) that two-thirds of the fathers who saw their child only monthly had contact with them by telephone and so on at least weekly and 45 per cent of fathers who saw their child only once every six months had contact with them at least once a fortnight. Adding together those who have either seen their child within the past two weeks or have contact with them in other ways once every two weeks, results in a total of 67 per cent of the fathers.

Table 6.11 Contact with children by telephone/letter/cards between visits

	%
At least once per week	62
At least once a fortnight	7
At least once a month	4
At least every three months	2
Once or twice a year	2
Less often	1
Not at all	23
N = 445	

Change in contact

The level of contact between non-resident fathers and their children is not necessarily static over time. Nearly half the fathers (44 per cent) had experienced changes in the contact arrangements since becoming a non-resident father, and the ones with the more stable arrangements tended to see their children more often. Fifty-two per cent of the fathers said that they now saw less of the children, and 45 per cent said they saw more of the children as a result of the change in the contact arrangement. The rest remained the same. The most common reason given for the reduction in contact was that the mother requested it (34 per cent), the child was too far away to see the father as often (15 per cent), and the child wanted to spend more time with their friends (10 per cent). There were also cases where the child asked for more contact (six), less contact (seven), and where a new partner asked for less contact (four) and more contact (one).

Children who visit their fathers

Eighty-four per cent of the fathers who saw their child more often than once a year, but who did not share care, had visits from the child. Whether or not there were visits did not seem to be affected by the living arrangements of the fathers. In 19 per cent of the cases where there was a visit to the father, the child could not or did not stay overnight, and there were a further six cases (1.5 per cent) where the visits involved a stay at the house of a relative or friend. Of those who stayed overnight, three-quarters of the children had their own bedroom to sleep in. Most of the fathers who had children to stay said that they managed without practical help – only 21 per cent said that they had help with baby-sitting, shopping, house-cleaning and so on from family or friends.

Fathers who visit children

Fifty-six per cent of the fathers visited their children and 31 per cent of these stayed overnight when they made their visit. Half of those who stayed, stayed in their ex-partner's house, 31 per cent stayed with relatives and friends, four cases in hotel and bed and breakfast and the rest with others. In some of these cases the child stayed with the father when he was not staying in the child's household, for example 21 per cent of those who stay with relatives and friends have the child to stay with them there.

Table 6.12 Activities

	% of responses	% of cases	N
Watch TV/video	20	62	277
Outings	12	37	166
Treats	9	28	126
Shopping	14	43	194
Cinema	3	10	46
Sport	6	19	84
Played	14	46	203
Visit relatives	10	30	135
Child had friend round to play	7	21	92
Other	6	19	86
All	101	315	1,409

Activities

The fathers were asked to think back to the last occasion that they had their child to visit or visited them, and were asked to list the things they did with them. The results are summarised in Table 6.12. The most common activity was watching TV or videos – nearly two-thirds of the cases – followed by playing, shopping and outings.

The fathers were asked whether they were involved in a set of activities that a resident father might be involved with. Of those with a school age child, 41 per cent visited school to attend parents evenings, 41 per cent helped with homework, 27 per cent picked up/dropped off at school, 24 per cent regularly taxied children around and 23 per cent baby-sat children under 14. Only 40 per cent engaged in none of these activities.

Emotional problems

Having contact with a child who is not resident may involve a certain amount of emotional trauma on the part of the child and the parents. Fathers were asked whether they found picking up the children or returning them to their mother after visits was distressing – 37 per cent of the fathers said that this was true for them, 30 per cent thought it was true for their children and 9 per cent for the child's mother, but 55 per cent thought that it was not true for any of them. The fathers were offered a list of typical traumas and asked whether they had experience of them. The results are summarised in Table 6.13. Only 23 per cent of the fathers had experienced none of these traumas and the most common experience was the father being upset – 43 per cent had

Table 6.13 Traumas associated with contact

	% of responses	% of cases	N
Child upset, does not want to leave mother	7	16	74
Child has nightmares	4	9	45
Child very clingy	13	31	145
Child has temper tantrums	10	23	111
Child does not want to return to mother	14	24	161
Child refuses to visit	4	9	45
You have been upset	18	43	207
You or ex-partner have shouted at each other	16	39	187
You have shouted at current partner	5	12	57
None of the above	10	23	110

experienced upset associated with contact, and 39 per cent had had experiences of shouting with their ex-partner. Over a third said that they had experience of the child not wanting to return to his or her mother and 9 per cent of the child refusing to visit them.

Relations with new partner

We found in the regression analysis of contact that those fathers who had repartnered and had a child living with them were less likely to have regular contact with their non-resident child. However, we also found that living with a new partner was associated with fathers having children to stay, and we found surprisingly few cases of the relationships between the child and new partners causing difficulty most (71 per cent) of the fathers said that their children got on with their new partner very well and 94 per cent very well or fairly well. In fact only two fathers said that the relationship was fairly bad or very bad.

Past partner

The fathers were asked whether they thought that their past partner was doing a good job bringing up their children – 39 per cent thought that they were doing a very good job and nearly 70 per cent a very good or fairly good job. It can be seen from Table 6.14 that they were much more likely to think that the mother was doing a good job when they had regular contact with the child. Most (75 per cent) of those who saw their child at least once a week thought that their partner was doing a very good or fairly good job, compared with only 45 per cent who saw their child less than once a year or never.

Table 6.14 Views about the performance of the resident parent

Partner doing a good job	At least once a week %	Once a fortnight %	Once a month %	Once a year %	Over one year or never %	All
Very good	45	37	34	27	30	39
Fairly good	30	31	27	30	15	29
Neither good nor bad	11	20	11	8	26	13
Fairly bad	9	6	18	18	15	11
Very bad	4	6	9	12	15	6
Don't know	1			5	(1)	2
All	290	86	44	66	27	514

Figures in brackets are numbers.

Relationship with children

The vast majority of the fathers thought that they got on well with their children – 84 per cent said that they got on very well, and a further 10 per cent fairly well. Only five fathers said that they got on very poorly. Not surprisingly, there was a strong association between the regularity of visits and quality of relationship. There was only one father who saw his child at least every week who said that they got on fairly poorly.

There were 442 fathers who thought their children were old enough to say whether they saw the father enough. Exactly half had said to their fathers that they did not see them as much as they would like to. There was no association between the frequency of contact and the children's view, possibly because children with more frequent contact were more likely to get the chance to express an opinion about the frequency of contact. Seventy-five per cent of the fathers with children who were old enough said that they thought that their children would like to see more of them than they did. Although they were more likely to say this if they had contact less than monthly, 70 per cent of those with contact at least weekly thought that their children would like to see them more than they do.

SUMMARY

In this chapter we have analysed the material in the sample survey relating to contact between the non-resident fathers and their children living with the mother in another household. The level of contact found in this sample was much higher than in studies of lone parents. It is probable that our sample is biased in favour of fathers who have contact with their non-resident child, though there may also be rather different perceptions of the meaning of contact between the caring and non-resident parent. With hindsight, seeing a child is not a satisfactory definition of contact. Contact is much more likely to be regular if there is an amicable relationship with the caring parent and if maintenance is being paid, but it is impossible to assess in which direction these relationships go. As we shall see, there is definitely a trade-off between contact and maintenance in the minds of non-resident fathers – they do not see why they should pay child support if their former partner obstructs contact with the child. Contact is much more regular if the father is in employment, if the child is young, if the father has no (new) children living in his household and if he lives near to the child. The relationship with the mother, which is critical to regular contact with the child, is more likely to be amicable if the father has not repartnered and does not have a new child in his household.

7 The fluidity of contact

INTRODUCTION

So far in this volume we have described how the men in this study became non-resident fathers, their present socio-economic circumstances and the patterns of contact they had with their non-resident children. In the preceding chapter the factors that influenced fathers' contact with their children were explored quantitatively. In this chapter we seek to enrich those findings from the insights gained from the first qualitative study of twenty in-depth interviews.

The twenty men were asked to describe the nature of their contact arrangements and any difficulties they faced, the input (or otherwise) of new partners in contact arrangements, and the nature of their relations with the children's mother as a co-parent. The characteristics of the fathers are described first before moving on to discuss the barriers they faced and the complexity of their contact arrangements, the influence of children in making their own arrangements, and how the wider kin network may have been involved in maintaining contact. In the second half of the chapter we will describe what it is like being a non-resident father and the difficulties faced in parenting children across different households. It is important to note that where the names of fathers or children are used, these are pseudonyms.

Characteristics of achieved sample

This sample comprised nineteen white men, and one Afro-Caribbean man. These men had very different life-styles and lived in both rural and urban locations throughout Britain. They had a broad range of occupations and varied levels of educational qualifications. All but one of the men in the sample had been married to their previous partners with whom they had children, although there had been no selection criteria to exclude cohabiting couples. In spite of the individual differences between these men, certain generalisations can be made about this group of respondents. They are a sample of older men: mean age 42.2 – with the youngest being 24, and three men clustering around age 50. The previously married men were emerging from long-term marriages, with the mean duration of marriages being eight and half years. Most of them lived near to their ex-partners and to their original birth families, and saw them on a regular basis. All the men who had been married had since divorced. Most men divorced very soon after separation – within seven to eight months – and within three years of separation all the men were divorced. All except three of the men were working, and had been employed in the same job for a good many years:

- three men were self-employed,
- three men were on disability benefits,
- fourteen men were employed in a variety of jobs.

Current family circumstances

Six of the men had remarried following separation from their former partners and three were cohabiting with new partners. Two of the men were living in households with their own children but no partner, four were living with other relatives, either their siblings or parents, and five men were living alone:

- six had remarried,
- three were cohabiting,
- one living with siblings,
- three with parents,
- two with children,
- five alone.

In total the twenty men in this sample had fathered forty-eight children from their past relationships, twenty-two of whom were girls. In addition they had a further thirteen stepchildren, some of whom were currently living in the men's households and some were not, plus a further six children born to current partners.

FINDINGS

The variety of contact arrangements

In five cases the fathers had *split residency* of their children from the same past family. Split residency is where some of the children born to the same parents lived with their fathers full-time and some with their mothers. As well as being non-resident fathers to some of their children, these five fathers were also the caring parent for other children. Thus they had complete responsibility for the children who lived with them and more limited responsibility for the children living with their ex-partners.

As well as these cases of split residency, six other fathers had *shared care* of their non-resident children. The definition of shared care used here was where a child (or all of the children) from the same family stayed overnight with their father at least 104 nights a year. This number of overnight stays was generally achieved by the child(ren) staying one night in the week, and then staying every weekend, or every other weekend. For the remaining nine fathers, two had no contact, two had limited contact because the children lived considerable distances away from their father, and the rest had fairly regular weekly contact:

- five men had split residency,
- six had shared care,
- five had weekly contact,
- two had limited contact because of distance,
- two had no contact.

Given that respondents were chosen for this qualitative study on the basis of them having contact, then the level of reported contact was high and all the men said they wanted to be involved in the care of their non-resident children, even the two fathers who had no contact. Why the two men without contact were not screened out during the process of selection never became clear. It could be that they were reluctant to give accurate information about contact in the quantitative survey as a result of accusations of child abuse; they had reported that court injunctions were in operation banning them from seeing their children.

In categorising contact as 'split residency', 'shared care' or 'regular contact', this implies that arrangements are somehow 'fixed', but this masks some of the complexity within individual families as well as the fluidity in contact arrangements, which change over time. For example, in cases of split residency where the children lived with their fathers, this generally followed a period of full-time residency with mothers. In two of these cases the change of residency of the children was prompted by difficult relations between the children and the mothers' new resident partners. Similarly, some arrangements could be very complex indeed. One of the fathers with split residency had his 11-year-old son from his previous marriage living with him full-time, while his two other children from that marriage lived with their mother 80 miles away. These two non-resident children came to stay with him in the school holidays. He also had his 10-month-old son from his current relationship living with him full-time, but the mother did not live with them even though his intimate relationship with her was ongoing. We also found that as children got older, they tended to make their own separate arrangements for spending time with their fathers. Fathers therefore did not necessarily see all of the children from the same family at the same time. This raises the question of how did the age of children affect contact arrangements? To explore this further, contact arrangements are described for the children as a whole group covering three different age bands: under 10 (when they would be most dependent), between 10 and 16 years of age (when children's independence is growing) and over 16 years (when arguably children are independent adults). The children of the two fathers without contact are excluded.

Ages of children and contact

Children under age 10

Nine children were under the age of 10. Six of these children regularly stayed overnight, and spent time with their fathers over holiday periods. In these cases, the children had a bedroom in their father's house, although sometimes they had to share this bedroom with a sibling. At the time of the interview, staying overnight had become somewhat routinised for these young children, in that the fathers reported it was no longer so strange or stressful. Once a routine had become established it was easier to move children between the mothers' and fathers' homes when they were young, because they had generally not yet established independent activities with their free time.

Only three of the fathers with children under the age of 10 did not have arrangements in place for the children to stay overnight regularly, though they did stay overnight occasionally. In all three cases the fathers lived close to their children, and they claimed they were actively involved in child-rearing. These arrangements for no, or minimal, overnight stays were agreements that had been negotiated with the mother for a variety of reasons; one father looked after his elderly parents, one of whom was bedridden, the other two felt it was better for their children to remain with their mothers, though all three expressed some regret about the lack of opportunity to spend more time with their children in this way.

Children aged between 10 and 16

Contact with children between the ages of 10 and 16 was still technically in place, but as the children were growing up and becoming more independent, the fathers found their contact arrangements were beginning to take second place after children's jobs, interests and friends. Three daughters in this age group had Saturday jobs that kept them very busy and gave them less time to spend with their fathers at the weekend. One of the fathers described the situation thus:

> They seem to be a lot more grown up these days. I mean my eldest, she's only 15 and she takes a two hour bus journey every Saturday morning to do a job, and then a two hour bus journey back. I mean my 11 year old, I mean to look at her, she looks about 14 or 15 and she acts like she is 14 or 15. I mean she's quite tall and big as well, but she's a lot older than what she is in years. I mean she goes off to Newcastle with her friend, but she's only 11. She'll get on the Metro and go to Newcastle with a friend.

Sometimes it was difficult for the fathers to get used to allowing their children to get on with their own lives.

> I get my nose put out of joint. I'm getting used to it now. Suddenly Dad's not required quite so much, you know erm. There's young men on the scene suddenly, instead of coming to me, she goes to Emma [friend]; and I'm getting used to it now, but it did put my nose out of joint a little bit.

Whether these experiences are any different for resident fathers is open to question.

Children over the age of 16

Children over the age of 16 all made independent arrangements to see their fathers. Several of the older children were living in flats of their own, and would drop in on their fathers regularly. For one father who suffered from manic depression, once his children got older he began to form a much closer relationship with them; they visited him regularly, but separately, at least once a week. However, another father found that as his children grew older he saw less of them. He described how he had imagined that when this two children had grown up they would decide to live with him, but this did not happen. He said:

> I've seen less of them, because I mean, they're studying now the majority of the time away, then when they do come back for holidays, they've got lots of things to do and so I've actually seen them less. I haven't wanted to nag them about coming to see me, so I think even in this . . . in this transition stage all parents have to go through, of sort of seeing their children go away and sort of, you know take their place in life and the parents probably miss the children as they are growing up at that stage. I would have felt that quite keenly too because I feel I happen to miss my children very much during their university periods.

According to the fathers, the age of children did not of itself appear to create much of a barrier in maintaining contact. The amount of contact could diminish or increase as children got older. Though it was possible that some fathers' relationships with children could improve the older children became, for others their children's increasing independence found them moving 'away from home' as they followed educational and other pursuits. There was therefore no guarantee that children's increasing age and ability to make independent arrangements with their fathers would increase contact time or frequency of visits. In the scheme of things these experiences might be exactly the same for resident fathers. However, there was one circumstance that could be said to be unique to non-residential fatherhood and that was the physical distance between their homes and those of their children. This could present considerable barriers for some in maintaining contact.

Distance

In only two of the eighteen cases where fathers had contact were children living some distance from their fathers' homes. However, the two cases were very different. In the first case, the father said that he was denied any contact with his three children for the first eighteen months after separating from his wife. He claimed that he had to go to court six times before he was given contact. At that time the judge agreed that the children should see their father once a month for a weekend – Friday to Sunday. The children were to be driven by their mother to a destination half-way between the two homes (which were 250 miles apart) where they would be met by their father. The visits went according to plan for the first few months but they ended because it was too stressful for all involved. Everyone was upset, and the children cried each time they had to leave their father. The mother had also failed repeatedly to make the rendezvous, arguing she could not get a lift to take the children. After that, contact broke down completely for five months, until the present system of visiting was established. Now the father visits his children at their mother's house every three months for a long weekend (he has to sleep on the sofa). His son also visits him, at his home in the holidays, but his two daughters have not visited his home for five years. These altered arrangements had only become possible because the father's relationship with his ex-wife had improved and he now found her supportive.

> She is helpful now. To be honest with you, she is probably the best she's ever been since we separated. She is slightly more than helpful, she can be really nice. I want to find a good way to sum it up. She is understanding. When my son wanted to come up here and stay with me there were no objections. He wanted to come up to London on his own on the coach. She was quite willing to pay for our son's trip to meet me. I met him in London and paid for his trip up to B. She puts me up when I stay there. We have nice friendly conversations on the phone every week.

Even though this arrangement was an improvement and was managed successfully, the father had to invest all his emotional energy in maintaining his relationships with his children (and his ex-wife). At times he questioned whether it was worth it. He described his feelings as:

> I told you I went through a few periods when I thought oh it's just not worth it, but you've got to persevere. I've had to make a real effort to see the children. It is hard and when I first made contact after those five months, after the split, I felt I had to recreate the friendship again, but I'd had about two years without really seeing them and in some way I was relying on it being like it was prior to that, but it wasn't. It totally took time. I had to talk to the children again. They were unsure how to treat me and had to learn how to treat me, because they hadn't seen me. The younger one, she was about three or four when she left. For her, she was really . . . it was like . . . who is this bloke, you know, and it was hard. . . . The two

older ones, because of their age when they left, they could still remember who I was, when I was part of the family unit . . . I don't feel like I am part of their lives.

For the second father whose children were living some distance from his home, he did not have to rely on the mother to provide him with accommodation. He either rented a cottage, or stayed in a bed and breakfast when he visited his sons. He preferred to take his two sons back to his own house, where his sons were brought up. However, as his two sons lived 500 miles away, this presented considerable practical difficulties and he only managed the trip home during school holidays and on the occasional weekend.

> Well it has been, it has been difficult because of the distance. And you know, the fact that I can only get so much time off. And then because of the distance it takes, you know, if I am going to bring them back here. It takes me two days travelling basically. To get them to and fro . . . and. . . . it's a long way for them to go as well you know. They get, they don't particularly enjoy the journey. Especially when they have just broken up from school and they are tired. It's a bit of a pain to them, but I, I see them every, I get to see them every school holiday, you know and the occasional weekend I go up.

There is no doubt that distance was a factor that made the maintenance of contact difficult – the quantitative work demonstrated that the longer the travelling time, the less likely fathers were to have regular contact. But the qualitative work shows that not only do fathers have to invest more time and more money, but they also have to cultivate a degree of emotional resilience, remain fairly flexible and keep negotiations open with mothers to maintain their commitment to visit their children. In addition, the need or preference to have children stay in their father's own home could add a further strain to contact arrangements when large travelling distances were involved. However, distance also made life harder for non-resident fathers in other ways. Both of the fathers complained that it was impossible to start any meaningful relationship with another woman while they were maintaining contact. Perhaps then it is not surprising that some fathers do not manage to sustain contact under these circumstances. The experiences of these two men highlight the importance of relationships with ex-partners for the continuance of contact, and this is now explored for the respondents as a whole.

Relationships with ex-partners

In this qualitative study as in others (Lund, 1987; Neale and Smart, 1997; Simpson *et al.*, 1995) not all of the fathers with contact managed to sustain good relationships with their ex-partners. To explore this further the fathers' co-parenting relationships with their ex-partners were examined along an axis of harmony or conflict. Obviously time played a part in the way ex-partners related to one another and we tried to capture this by asking fathers to describe their relations with their ex-partners at the point of separation and how they were now. Fathers' current relationships were therefore categorised as harmonious (Table 7.1) or conflictual (Table 7.2). It is noteworthy that this part of the interview was the most stressful; in reliving the past, the fathers could be overcome with feelings of loss, grief and anger and for some these feelings were not reconciled.

Reconciled or still angry?

Overall, at the time of the interview, ten of the fathers had settled or reasonable co-parenting relationships with their ex-partners and these were categorised as 'harmonious'. Eight had conflictual relations and the two fathers without contact had no relationship with their ex-partners.

Of these ten harmonious relationships, four either had amicable or indifferent feelings towards their ex-partners at the time of separation, while another four gave muted descriptions about their feelings at the time of separation, saying their relationships with their ex-partners were 'tense' or that they felt 'hurt'. For seven of these eight, current relations tended not to be described in a positive manner but rather in terms of absence of conflict. They either 'got on fine', or things were 'alright' or things were 'settled'. Only one said his ex-partner was 'very helpful'. For these eight, the quality of co-parenting relationships seemed quite stable over time, neither improving greatly nor deteriorating (see Table 7.1).

In contrast, the other two fathers with harmonious relations at the time of interview had experienced considerable improvements in their relationships from the point of separation. They described their feelings at the time of the breakup as being full of 'hate' and wanting to 'kill' the mother. Yet now, one of them was very positive about his relationship, describing his ex-partner as 'understanding' and 'helpful'. The other remained uncertain and sceptical, saying that his ex-partner was 'nice to him' only if she wanted something. It seemed that these two had much higher levels of anger and animosity to overcome and it was against this backdrop that their relationships had improved.

Table 7.1 Change in relationships for fathers with harmonious co-parenting
relationships

Relationships at the point of separation	Relationships at interview	Total showing improvement
8 Amicable or indifferent	'Fine'; 'settled'; 'alright'	2 only
2 Very hostile	'Helpful' (1)	
	'Uncertain' (1)	
Total 10 fathers		

Although relationships were generally harmonious, they were not exceptionally friendly and could be summed up as polite but distant. This was in contrast to the eight fathers who had conflictual co-parenting relationships.

The fathers with conflictual relationships seemed to be locked into a cycle of bitterness and revenge and they maintained high levels of anger and resentment against their ex-partners. Unlike the harmonious co-parenting group, these fathers with conflictual relationships exhibited many different permutations of changes in relationships. Two fathers started off with reasonable relationships but these had deteriorated over time; two other fathers' relationships went from 'bad to worse'; three more had 'very difficult' relationships in the beginning that had not changed over time, and one father said his relationship had improved slightly from the point of separation. However, this improvement was couched in terms of the relationship moving from being highly argumentative to a complete absence of communication. This father described the current situation as follows:

> Well I don't see her. I just pull up outside the house, [and] daughter comes out.

Therefore although all these fathers had conflictual co-parenting relationships at the time of interview, in one case this was actually an improvement from before, while in two others relations had deteriorated since separation (see Table 7.2).

A variety of reasons were proffered by fathers as to why their relationships were conflictual, but no one reason was common to all fathers. The reasons included:

- the mother's continued resentment at the father's infidelity;
- the mother's perception that the father was an irresponsible parent;

- the father's mental illness – in one case the father suffered from manic depression;
- constant arguments and disagreements;
- the father feeling 'shoved out' of the children's lives; and
- mothers' developing new partnerships (but interestingly not fathers' developing new partnerships).

Table 7.2 Change in relationships for fathers with conflictual co-parenting relationships

Relationships at the point of separation	Relationships at interview	Total showing deterioration	Total showing improvement
2 'Reasonable'	'As bad as you can', 'Fairly hostile now'	2 only	1 only
2 'Hostile' or 'bitter'	'Very hostile'		
3 'Very difficult' or 'very bitter'	Remained the same		
1 'Full of arguments'	Arguments ceased as communication stopped		
Total 8 fathers			

Overall, eighteen of the fathers still had some kind of relationship with their ex-partners, but having a good or reasonable relationship at the time of separation was no guarantee that things would continue that way. Conversely very hostile relationships at the point of separation could improve over time. According to the respondents one factor in particular that affected relationships and contact arrangements was the mother developing a new partnership, yet fathers felt their own new partnerships were not so influential. The influence of these new partnerships is now explored.

Mothers' new partnerships

What became clear from the accounts of some of these eighteen men, was that relationships with ex-partners sometimes had to endure frequent changes in family structures as new partners arrived and later departed from the mothers' households. For example, in three cases the mothers moved directly into another relationship at the point of separation. Two of these relationships had subsequently failed and in one of these cases the mother had married for a third time. The fathers reported that the children's relationships with the mothers' new partners were a source of constant tension. This could place the non-resident fathers in a difficult position in regard to their own relationships with their children. For example, Dave had witnessed the failure of his ex-wife's second marriage and was now caught up in the difficulties his children were experiencing in her third marriage. He described the situation thus:

> Yes it is difficult. I am finding increasingly now that when they have been with me at the weekends. Because they say he [stepfather] is so strict at home, I am finding it difficult to get them to go back. I have a lot of tears on Sundays. Sam, the oldest of the boys was refusing to go back. I managed to get him in the car in the end in tears and he ran straight into the house at the other end saying he was going to pack his stuff and leave. The difficulty I am finding is that I want them to understand that they can come and live with me if things become impossible at the other end but I don't want to encourage that. I don't want to put them in a position where they are being tugged.

Later he went on to say:

> I felt completely useless when Sam was in tears saying he wasn't gonna go home. Do you encourage it and say 'Yes Sam OK, OK you can come and live with me.' Or do you say, 'no get back in there kid. You've got to sort out the battle yourself cos I can't help you.'

From Dave's perspective he had to watch from the sidelines as the mother's relationships with new partners unfolded (the converse is also true for mothers watching non-resident fathers' relationships unfold). But Dave's story highlights how this could present difficulties for him as the non-resident father; perhaps there were difficulties too for some children if they feel forced into making a choice as to which parent they should live with. His 16-year-old daughter (one of four children from that marriage) had already moved in with Dave, apparently as a result of conflicts with the stepfather. In contrast, fathers' new partners were not seen as having any effect on fathers' relationships with their non-resident children.

Fathers' new partnerships

The fathers who had developed new cohabiting relationships (including those who had remarried) were adamant that their new partners were not involved in contact arrangements with children. These women were also ascribed a minimal role in terms of their interaction with the fathers' children – that they would act like friends only and that the fathers retained full parental responsibility. Perhaps the new partners, had we been able to interview them, would have reported their involvement with these children rather differently. This does not mean to say, however, that fathers' new partners had no effect on co-parenting relationships, but rather it was of a different order to the effect mothers' new partners had on relationships. For example, the men reported that their new partnerships often aroused feelings of jealousy in their ex-partners and this created tensions in co-parenting relationships. A new cohabitation, or a new birth in the father's family, was often the catalyst for a renewed period of troubled relations with the ex-partner, whereas mothers' new partners were presented as being problematic primarily in terms of their relationships with the fathers' children. This could simply reflect the fact that non-resident children were spending more time with their stepfathers as they lived in the same household. Resident 'stepfathers', therefore, may be more involved in parenting than non-resident 'stepmothers' and thus the opportunities for difficulties arising between stepfathers and children would be greater.

Some of the other respondents who lived alone (or with their children) were aware of this potential for conflict attached to new partnerships and this inhibited them from cohabiting or remarrying. For example, four of the men living alone did have ongoing relationships with women, but had made the decision that life was easier without cohabitation. One of these fathers, who had split residency of his children (his daughter Amy lived with him and his three sons did not), described the difficulties thus:

> Not that we wouldn't like to [live together], but I'm determined to keep space for my children. That, that's paramount. I'll always do that, so there is no question of us moving in together. Not that we wouldn't like it, but it would be difficult with Amy and the other children. Tension would come in; Amy wouldn't get on with Jenny's [girlfriend's] children. So if we were living there it would be very difficult. I think the children need their own space. My boys feel that.

Accommodating new partnerships was not always easy, especially if the new partner had children of her own. Therefore some of the men in this sample preferred to sacrifice the opportunity for a cohabiting relationship in order to protect their space and time with their non-resident children.

Overall, the fathers' relationships with ex-partners were very complex. Not only were they rooted in feelings and conflicts surrounding the causes of separation, which may or may not have been resolved, but they were subject to constant challenges and pressures as both parents developed new partnerships and second families. Most importantly, the development and possible failure of subsequent partnerships demonstrates the dynamic nature of relationships and the fluidity of family structure both within and across these parents' distinct households. Perhaps only a few people – women, children and men – have the ability to manage this fluidity and resultant ambiguity in family relationships without conflict. As Dave said:

> You have to stop yourself despite what you know. Despite what you are trying to do, you have to stop the sarcastic comments. Because despite yourself they are there under the surface. It's difficult sometimes. I don't know how you do it, it's so silly.

In comparison, the fathers' relationships with their families of origin were much more stable (see Chapter 3) and we specifically intended to investigate whether extended families provided a social network that would assist them in the parenting of their children following separation.

Extended family

We found that thirteen of the fathers in this sample still lived near to their brothers/sisters and parents, and most of these fathers saw their parents at least once a week (this was comparable to the quantitative data presented in Chapter 3). It was quite common, for the fathers who visited their parents more than once a week, to have at least one meal a week in their old family home. A pattern described by three of the fathers was to call in on their mothers on the way home from work – if there was food around they might eat and then go home. Most often, the frequent visits were described in terms of just calling in to see if their mother wanted anything, or to see if their fathers wanted to go out to the pub. The fathers who saw their parents and siblings more than once a week said they were emotionally very close to them.

The relationships with parents were good enough for seven of the fathers to have moved back home to live with their parents, at least for a short time after their relationships had broken down. At the time of the interview four of them were still living at home. One of these four was living in the parental home with two of his brothers, who were also convalescing after failed marriages. He also had five sisters living locally whom he saw several times a week. 'If you take one of us, you take the lot', was how he summed up his feelings about his family.

In four cases the fathers' mothers played a crucial role in maintaining the fathers' relationships with their children, especially in the early days of separation when tempers were frayed and all were under stress. Indeed two of the fathers had gone abroad for a few months following separation and in both these cases their mothers had stepped into the breach, and maintained the link for their grandchildren. It is worth examining the influence of grandmothers in more depth through a case study – Terry.

Terry

At the time of interview Terry was happily married to his second wife Barbara and had a second family. Terry has now settled down and is an active and committed father to his children from both of his families, but it was not always like this. Terry and Julie married when she got pregnant when she was still at school; she was 16 and he was 18. They very quickly had another child and Terry became more and more disenchanted with his life and responsibilities, as did Julie. He finished his apprenticeship, but he had begun to realise what he had missed by settling down so young. He decided to leave Julie. He moved back in with his parents for a short time, but this proved impossible because Terry said he got on very badly with his father, who was ashamed of his son for running out on his family. Terry left and went to live in the south of France, and then he moved on to Amsterdam. He was away on and off for a few years, keeping in touch with his mother and his daughters only by postcard. He came back for short visits, but he said he wanted excitement and action abroad. During this time his mother provided a vital link with his first family. She had his daughters to stay regularly, and kept him informed of their progress, and kept up a relationship with Julie. Eventually Terry got tired of travelling and came home. Again for a while he lived with his parents. While he was there, his mother would arrange for his daughters to spend the weekend with them, and make sure Terry was there.

> They'd stay at me Mum's, and me Mum'd have em down in the week um, in fact if it hadn't been for me Mum a lot of the time I probably wouldn't have bothered seeing 'em you know. It was me Mum who brought them down . . . made sure I was there when they were there kind of thing.

In Terry's case, his links with the children were made and maintained by his mother, who continued her involvement with her grandchildren, and forced her son to retain his commitment to them. Now twelve years on, he is able to acknowledge her help. Terry admitted that he would have lost contact with his children, that he was young and selfish, and virtually abandoned them when he went abroad for two years. His relationship with his daughters is not without its problems now; one is a difficult teenager, who blames her father for his neglect, but he sees her regularly and is trying to make things up to her as best he can.

What was unforeseen at the beginning of the study was the importance of the family of origin in sustaining the father's involvement with his children. For some of these respondents, the extended family played an important part in helping the father with his obligations to his children, on a practical level in terms of providing a home, and on an emotional level in terms of support.

Grandmothers in particular could be 'invisible' facilitators in the maintenance of contact and fathers' relationships with their children.

So far we have described how various factors work to inhibit or aid fathers' contact with their children, but we have not described what it is like being a non-resident father and the difficulties faced in continuing to parent children across different households. It is to this we now turn in the second half of this chapter.

BEING A NON-RESIDENT FATHER

We wanted to find out from these men what it was like being a non-resident father. One of the problems, according to Richards and Dyson (1982), is that the behaviour of fathers is measured against the behaviour of mothers with children; there is no separate agenda for fathers. In this view, the role of the father has not been disentangled from the role of the mother. Yet following divorce and separation the fathers must learn to operate as a parent on their own with their children – at least, that is, without the physical presence of the mother. In that sense the role of the non-resident father is more like the role of the mother, in that the men might assume all responsibilities and all executive functions. Therefore when exploring what it is like being a non-resident father, we will consider two things: first, what it was like for these men to be an active parent on a part-time basis during contact visits, and second, how did the men manage as parents alone – that is without the presence of the children's mothers? As already highlighted, two of the men did not have contact with their children and these two are excluded from this part of the analysis.

Fathering alone?

The fathers saw their relationships with their children in terms of spending time together, doing things together, playing games rather than spending money – shopping and buying treats. Doing things together was one of the most common responses from fathers, when asked what they did with their children.

> Yes I like playing with them and reading them stories and lots and lots of stuff. . . . They love coming to me and I love having them. We do a lot together and we go to . . . we play on computers a lot and I am always taking them out and doing things. Sam is very into Scouts and playing football and all sorts of things like that. They always want to bring their friends over here as well. Little Matthew more now is bringing friends here as well, which I like.

It was not all fun and games, however; the men were keen to point out that life carried on more or less 'normally', with arguments and household chores to be done. Additionally all eighteen of the men complained about the limitations imposed upon them by the extra costs involved in paying child support and supporting a separate house. Limited resources meant that they could not entertain their children all the time by paying for expensive recreational activities outside the home. One father recounted not only how his son had understood this but how the father had found this helpful.

> The only thing in my favour is that I can sit and talk to the children. They are at an age when they can understand. I think the son has helped me a lot. The son, he wants to come and spend time with me. It's his choice. He wants to, when I've explained to him now it's cost lots of money. He will just sit there in the house and not want to go out. He doesn't need to go out. When he comes up I do take him out, it's nice. It's nice that he's got me included in his life, in his future.

From this father's account it appears that the son's apparent understanding of the financial constraints had created a sense of relief and reassurance for the father. The father knew that the son wanted to be with him regardless of the father's ability to pay for outside entertainment. Even though there were echoes of these non-resident fathers acting as 'Disney time fathers' or acting like 'Father Christmas' (Hess and Camara, 1979), some were also settled into a more mundane routine of parenting.

Becoming a non-resident father – and therefore parenting alone – was also a very positive experience for some of these fathers and was actually seen as an improvement in their relationships with their children. They made concerted efforts to get to know their children very well and they had to learn to do things with them, rather than just being the mother's 'deputy'. This was challenging to the fathers who had functioned with the mother as a parent, rather than taking the lead in the relationship with the children, and some of these fathers found that the new role needed rethinking.

> I found the . . . my separation um . . . hugely undermining of my role as father . . . um because even though as I say, one did all sorts of nice things with the kids at the weekend and they were very good and nice about wanting to come and see me . . . but when they . . . I mean frankly the whole role of father changes . . . the very sort of fundamental nature of fatherhood, you know, being apart, I mean, you're forced to rethink it over and you probably just accept it as a role. I mean, I'm not saying I was a terribly good father before but in some ways my fathering had to improve because I had to improve it, I mean, my daughter now, sometimes sort of jokes and also teases me about her sort of memory of me as a father, and this was this bloke at the end of the garden cutting the lawn . . . I did work long hours, so I wasn't available till later in the week, um and . . . but I was always there at weekends and obviously her image is an exaggeration but it's funny that I should even . . . I didn't seek to deny it.

Fathering full-time on a part-time basis?

Although fathers saw their new parenting responsibilities positively for most of the time, there were times when not being constantly with the child proved difficult. Obviously, the situation is very different depending on the amount of contact experienced by the father and his children. Visits for an afternoon once every now and then are very different from regular overnight or weekend contact. But the fathers who saw their children mainly at weekends experienced all the complexities of fulfilling the father role alongside adjusting to the 'on/off' nature of their parenting. They had sole responsibility for feeding, washing, amusing, teaching, playing with, shopping, visiting relatives and all practical aspects of child-rearing at the weekend and thus the weekends could be very hectic. But there was also an added sense of urgency where the fathers felt they had to make up for lost time while simultaneously trying to lead an 'ordinary' family life.

Things erm, become more urgent. That you have an agenda at the weekend. And if you have to talk something through, if you want to talk something through with any of them. Whether you're in the mood or not. Whether they are in the mood or not. It sometimes has to be done. So you've got less choice over the moment. And also of the domestic side of things. There's my little boy still wets the bed, so you've the washing of sheets and pyjamas at the weekend, and if they . . . oh all manner of things you do. You're likely to be so busy so you don't have periods of inactivity, which I think you have in a situation where they are there all the time and you can take your time over things.

Between visits from their children, these fathers had to carry on with their own interests and pursue their own lives, and for those who were single men this created a sense of discontinuity in their role as fathers. This is the continuity/discontinuity that is evident for non-resident fathers. The continuity consisted of maintaining a relationship with the child following separation, but to do so on a fluctuating basis whereby the father had to adopt two different life-styles, one during the week and the other at weekends. The ten fathers who had not repartnered and had been acting as a lone parent at the weekend felt the transitions between the two separate parts of their lives more acutely. The child had been the total focus of the father's attention, and then the child had gone. One father had this to say:

It gets very lonely. All of a sudden, this whirlwind of energy and enthusiasm is no longer there. Often you find yourself looking for things to do. When your child is not there you have nothing to do, because you are constantly entertaining him when he is.

The fathers who devoted every weekend to their children were happy to do this, and they took their responsibilities very seriously, even in some cases denying themselves social time with friends.

I'm the responsibility, she's my responsibility should I say. I'd rather spend time with her than go out. Well I finish work at half past five and it takes ten minutes to get here, so it's just after 5.30 and she goes at 6 pm on Sunday. Well when the weather's bad now so she just stays in and plays all sorts of games, and what not – painting and writing. When it's decent weather we usually go for a day out on the Sunday – anywhere – parks – the zoo – she loves animals, so we go to the zoo or safari park.

However, while the men appeared devoted to their children and committed to continuing to parent them, some found it very stressful at times. One particular problem was disciplining or controlling children's behaviour during contact visits. Half of the fathers said that they suffered from guilt because of the failure of their relationship and its impact on their children, and as a result were at times too lenient. They allowed their children to get away with behaviour that they, as fathers, felt was unacceptable.

> When I see her, whereas if she were here all the time every day, obviously I'd go 'give it a rest Kylie' not abuse . . . but you know what I mean. You can't take it day in day out . . . an' because I only see her on them two days I will say 'What d'yr want; what do y'r want?' all the time and do it for her. So I have to concentrate the week's events into two days.

Because some fathers found weekend parenting a strain, at times they could also find themselves feeling very angry.

> We're very close. With me, me Mum, and Charlotte [daughter]; and it's a fine line between love and hate. I go to me Mum [and say] 'I hate her, I bloody hate her [hate the daughter]', and then it gets close to time to go back and you think and you take her back and it's all quiet again.

Having weekend visits was quite difficult to adjust to. On the one hand the fathers could devote themselves fully to their children during weekend visits, which was generally felt to be a positive experience, but the downside of this was the sudden absence of their children in their lives midweek. On the other hand having the children to stay full-time at weekends was stressful for some as they found their children's behaviour difficult to cope with. Additionally, although these fathers were parenting their children without the physical presence of the mother, this did not mean that mothers had no influence on the father's parenting. The influence of mothers, however, was diffuse and indirect. The mere existence of the mother as another parent was problematic as it could engender feelings of parental competition.

Parental competition?

The younger fathers in this qualitative sample were more critical of their ex-wives, and also more confident in their own fathering abilities than the older fathers. They certainly did not see their role in terms of just being the mother's back-up. These fathers had their own ideas on bringing up a healthy child, which included providing a good diet (not just McDonald's) and a good standard of hygiene, and sometimes they felt themselves to be better parents than the mother. Nigel, a young father of 24, had this to say:

> I don't think she's as good a mother as I am a father. Nothing really – just little things. You can pick her up [his daughter] and she's dirty, just generally grubby. Um she smells of smoke, very often she has been in a smoky room. She'll have a cough one weekend when I pick her up. So we only have two days for the cough to clear up and she goes back with a tickle . . . and we pick her up next weekend and she'll still have a cough, so she's not been to the doctor or anything. It's not as if I say it's abuse or neglect . . . it's slight neglect really it's the little things.

Another young father, Stan, felt he was more attentive towards his child than his ex-wife whom he accused of being interested only in horses. Consequently Stan felt he had a stronger relationship with his daughter than his ex-wife, and now at the age of 15 he said his daughter was considering coming to live with him full-time.

> My wife got jealous of my relationship with my eldest daughter – proper Daddy's girl sitting on my knee and that. I spent a lot of time with them. The wife always worked – she would go out to work as soon as I got home, so I spent a lot of time with them. When I was home I'd do everything – get their tea, put them to bed – get them up in the morning, take them to school on me bike . . . I always got on very well with the children. My eldest daughter looks just like me . . . is just like me . . . if she has something to say, she says it . . . that's like me, that's the way they've been brought up. So she doesn't get on well down there [her mother's house].

Jensen (1995) has argued that at a time when some men are becoming more emotionally attached to their children they are simultaneously becoming more physically detached, as they have to work increasingly long hours to support their families. For non-resident fathers it seems that this paradox of closeness and distance is exaggerated further. They are more physically detached from their children in terms of the reduction of daily interactions with them, but potentially find themselves having stronger emotional attachments as they develop a new one-to-one relationship in the context of parenting alone. As some non-resident fathers in this sample have shown, their increasing identification with parenthood created an element of parental competition as time with children was scarce; thereby the man's self-identity as a father could also be threatened. However, this was not the only tension created as a result of shared parenthood. Some of these children appeared to have quite different rules of conduct in each of their parents' households and this had potentially negative consequences for the fathers' relationships with their children.

One father had this to say about his 8-year-old son from his previous marriage, which had ended very acrimoniously:

> He's the only child of a very very obsessive mother and so positively adored, loved and spoilt, but also tiresome very spoilt child and I hope he doesn't become alienated from other kids his age because of it, and become a sad character. Fortunately so far, there is no sign of it and his integration seems to be very good. I have felt some resentment to him lately, because he has come to expect when he comes round here for me to play with him; he expects me to play with him and for some reason got quite stroppy about it; he didn't want me to sit down or have a cup of tea; so it's really been quite a strain sometimes. And I must admit, the weekends I am not having him, I sort of look forward to as a relief that I haven't got to spend my time with looking after a boisterous 8-year-old.

He went on to say:

> His table manners are appalling, why doesn't he ever help out with meals? I mean it it's ridiculous, really you know he should behave better than this.

Another father who had weekly visits from his children expected that they would contribute to the running of the household as they got older. This father, who had three daughters, explained how he had pressured his girls to help in the home, with much protesting from them. He complained that his ex-wife did not make any demands on his daughters, and did not expect them to help.

> Well, to me, she does everything for them and I mean everything. I mean just washing the dishes, the arguments I had with that. You know, I mean, I say 'Anybody washing the dishes?' It was 'Oh no we don't wash dishes' and that. I said 'Do you do anything?' She

said 'No'. She just does everything for them. Well I don't think that is right. They should be made to chip in, you know. Not earn their keep, I mean, well you know, sort of help out or something like that.

Therefore overall being a non-resident father had many facets, some negative and some positive. It is hard to say how many of these facets concern parenting in general and therefore are experienced by all parents – disciplining children, for example, is something all parents have to negotiate. But it seemed there was an added tension in non-resident parenting as the children's unruly or difficult behaviour could be blamed upon the other parent (the mother). Similarly fathers may have found themselves developing closer relationships with their children, but this could create an element of parental competition as the fathers vied with the mother for the children's loyalty and affection. According to these men, however, the most critical difference between being a father and being a non-resident father, was the loss of continuity. This was not a big dramatic loss, for the eighteen of these fathers who saw their children; but the loss of continuity reflected the absence of frequent and daily interactions that would normally take place when co-resident with children on a full-time basis. As a result of not being around, the fathers treated seemingly trivial events with far more importance than if they had been in permanent residence. But the loss of continuity was also seen nostalgically, as to what might have been if the father had stayed living with the children. Perhaps this sense of loss was due to something far more abstract, the loss of possibility. Though fathers expressed their sense of loss in similar terms, for some this was juxtaposed with the possibility for greater involvement with their children than they had during their partnership, whereas for others, particularly the two men without contact, the loss was absolute. It is appropriate to add a note of caution here. The two fathers without contact had court injunctions against them forbidding them to see their children as a result of suspected child sex abuse. This provides a salutary reminder that when discussing contact, the welfare of children must remain paramount. Non-resident fathers' contact with children may not be desirable in all cases, no matter what the sense of loss.

SUMMARY

The ages of children had an influence on the nature of contact, in that as they got older they could spend relatively more, or even relatively less, time with their fathers. Similarly, a large distance between the father's household and that of the children could disrupt contact to such an extent that the fathers' could question whether the effort was 'worth it'.

Even so, children and grandmothers were themselves major actors in maintaining contact and new partners were not (at least as reported by these men). Though some ex-partners were seen as being instrumental in reducing fathers' relationships, others, though fewer, were described as helpful. New partnerships could create tensions in relationships, particularly when the mothers' new partners were acting as 'stepfathers'. Competition with mothers for children's affection and time could also arouse tension, as did different disciplinary codes across parents' households.

Quite apart from these inhibitors and facilitators of contact, these respondents were also fulfilling a number of roles as fathers. Fatherhood has previously been conceptualised as a status with a variety of different roles, for example provider, disciplinarian and companion. As Daly (1995) comments, although (resident) fathers are actively engaged in shaping their roles, this is constrained by the structural context within which their fathering takes place. Clearly this is highly pertinent to non-resident fathers, where the whole structural arrangement in terms of housing and time spent with children and the whole emotional institution of the two-parent family have altered dramatically. The evidence from the fathers in this sample highlighted a number of varied difficulties in adjusting to their role as a non-resident father. These included:

- rethinking their role as a father – particularly as a lone parent during contact visits;
- measuring their parenting style against the mother in a competitive manner and therefore often being critical of the mother as a parent;
- deciding upon when and how to discipline children – concerns here over being:
  - too lenient,
  - teaching children manners and being unclear about expectations of children's participation in chores around the father's household, and
  - upholding standards of children's conduct that seem in contradiction with the standards set by the mother;
- adjusting to the immediacy of children's needs (both physical/practical and emotional needs) in concentrated bursts over weekend visits; and
- adjusting to and grieving for the absence of children in their daily lives.

Even with these difficulties, the fathers with contact said that the worst thing that could happen to them was losing contact with their children altogether.

What we have not discussed here is the possible link between emotional and financial relationships with children (or contact and maintenance), which is covered in the subsequent chapters on maintenance.

8 Child support: Who pays?

INTRODUCTION

The issue of child support[14] has become probably the most salient policy issue affecting non-resident parents since Margaret Thatcher declared:

> No father should be able to escape from his responsibility and that is why the government is looking for ways of strengthening the system for tracing an absent father and making the arrangements for recovering maintenance more effective.
>
> (Text of the National Children's Homes' George Thomas Society Lecture, 17 January, 1990)

The new interest in child support arose partly as a result of the increase in the numbers of lone parents and their dependence on benefits, partly from a more fundamentally moral view that biological parents should be responsible for their children throughout their lives, and partly from the knowledge derived from research that existing maintenance awards through the courts were low, irregularly paid and often not reviewed over time. The Bradshaw and Millar (1991) survey found that only 29 per cent of lone parents at any one time were receiving regular payments from a non-resident father, with a mean payment per child of £16 per week. When the White Paper 'Children Come First' was published in 1990, benefit savings and increased incentives for lone parents to join the labour force were added to the objectives of the reforms of child support. In the Second Reading of the Child Support Bill the hope was also expressed that enforcing the obligation to pay maintenance might persuade fathers to retain their marital and paternal duties and be less inclined to conceive children outside marriage.

The Child Support Act 1991 was intended to sweep away the old arrangements for maintenance, which had been based on a dual system through the courts and in the 'liable relative procedures' in social security law and administration. A Child Support Agency was to be established with powers to assess and enforce child support payments, using a standard, and supposedly simple, formula. All 'absent' parents were to be covered by the new scheme, whether or not their former partner was dependant on social security benefits, and whether or not they had made an agreed settlement before the passage of the Act.[15]

This is not the place to review in detail the history of the débâcle of child support since the Child Support Agency began operations in April 1993. Suffice it to say that it is probably one of the worst examples of social policy making in modern history. It is widely agreed that the Act contained some fundamental flaws – including its retrospective nature and the absence of a disregard for those on Income Support. The formula was too complicated for the parties involved to understand, and at the same time there was no scope for varying it to take account of exceptional circumstances or special needs. The Act was very poorly scrutinised by Parliament – there was general support for the principle of the Act and not enough attention paid to the detail. The implementation of the Act by the Child Support Agency was a fiasco, with inadequate computer systems, poor management and ill-prepared staff. The result was huge delays and backlogs, inaccurate assessments, incompetent or non-existent enforcement, which has all resulted in confusion, misery (including some suicides, NACSA claims) and a general loss of confidence in the Agency by both lone parents and non-resident fathers. After five years of operation, one amending Act, endless changes in regulations, the departure of two chief executives, five parliamentary select committee inquiries and repeatedly critical reports from the National Audit Office, the child support system is failing to deliver on all its objectives. Non-compliance and collusion are thought to be epidemic and according to CSA annual accounts 1997/98 arrears amount to about £600 million. A dual system has become re-established: the child support system for lone parents on means-tested benefits and other arrangements through lawyers and the courts for other people. The proportion of lone parents receiving regular child support is scarcely different from what it was under the old system, and the level of payments, which have fallen as a result of changes to the formula, are also not much greater (taking into account inflation since 1989). It is arguable and argued by the National Association for Child Support Action (NACSA – previously the Network Against the Child Support Act) that if account is taken of the costs of administering the CSA, then the savings to the public purse have been minuscule or non-existent over the old system.

The new Labour Government is in the process of reviewing the Child Support Act. There is a strong body of political opinion, including the commitment of the Liberal Democrat Party, to abandoning the Act and returning to a court-based, or at least judicial system, that allows for more flexible, individualised justice than the formula-driven scheme.

The findings of this research

In this chapter we concentrate on the issue of who pays child support, drawing on the results of the sample survey. In Chapter 9 we continue by exploring the level of formal and informal support provided by non-resident fathers. In Chapter 10 we draw on the sample survey and the second qualitative study to present findings of fathers' experiences of the Child Support Agency. Then finally in Chapters 11 and 12 we draw on the qualitative material to explore non-resident fathers' views about their financial obligations. Note that the findings presented here on child maintenance relate only to the most recent previous partnership in which fathers had children, and not to all past relationships in cases where fathers had multiple past relationships involving children.

Who pays child support?

The non-resident fathers were asked two distinct questions about money payments: first, whether they now or had ever made regular or occasional payments for child maintenance; second, whether they now make money payments for child maintenance. We found that 77 per cent had paid at some time and 57 per cent were currently paying. There is considerable disparity between these fathers' reports of maintenance paid and that reported by lone parents in other studies. Bradshaw and Millar (1991) found that only 40 per cent of lone mothers had ever received maintenance payments and only 30 per cent were currently (in 1989) receiving them. Marsh, Ford and Finlayson (1997) found in their national survey of lone parents (including lone fathers) that only 30 per cent received maintenance in 1994.

As with the disparity we have already explored in relation to contact, some further analysis was conducted on the Bradshaw and Millar data to examine to what extent this disparity could be explained. In the Bradshaw and Millar (1991) study maintenance payments varied by the employment status of the fathers. Thus where lone mothers said the father was employed, just under half received maintenance compared with only 8 per cent of those whose former partners were unemployed. The rates of unemployment of fathers in the Bradshaw and Millar study (where the status was known by the mother) were higher than in this study; some 48 per cent of lone mothers' former partners were employed, compared with 66 per cent of non-resident fathers in this study who were employed. Similarly the proportion of lone mothers receiving maintenance varied considerably according to their previous marital status. The ex-married lone mothers were much more likely to be receiving maintenance – some 31 per cent of the ex-married compared with 18 per cent of the ex-cohabiting and only 13 per cent of the ex-single were receiving maintenance at the time of the study.

Of the ex-married fathers in this sample, 66 per cent of the divorced and 61 per cent of the previously married but separated fathers claimed to be paying maintenance at the time of the study. Only 39 per cent of the ex-cohabiting fathers were paying and 48 per cent of the never married/never cohabited (they made up only 10 per cent of the whole sample) fathers claimed to be paying maintenance currently. Lone mothers in the Bradshaw and Millar survey had not repartnered (by definition) but where the fathers in this study knew the partnership status of the mother 57 per cent of the mothers had repartnered. If we restrict the analysis to those who are still known to be lone mothers then we find that fathers were paying maintenance to 62 per cent of these. So as with contact, when we control for some of the differences between non-resident fathers in this sample and the non-resident fathers of the children of lone mothers, some of the gap but by no means all of it is closed.

There remain two possible reasons for this discrepancy: first, this sample is not representative and is biased in favour of non-resident fathers who pay maintenance (it is possible that Bradshaw and Millar is also is biased though this is unlikely given that Marsh, Ford and Finlayson (1997) have confirmed their findings on maintenance); second, non-resident fathers are exaggerating the extent to which they pay maintenance, and lone mothers are diminishing the extent to which they receive it, as it may be in their interest to do so. There is no incentive for lone mothers in receipt of means-tested benefits to declare that they receive maintenance, because as there is no disregard for those on Income Support, they risk losing their benefits; over three-quarters of lone mothers are dependent on one or other means-tested benefits. Non-resident fathers, on the other hand, stand to gain by declaring maintenance payments, as paying would enhance their reputation as responsible fathers.

Fathers' individual characteristics

Table 8.1 compares the characteristics of fathers by the payment of maintenance. Particularly striking was the difference in the employment

Table 8.1 Payment of maintenance, by fathers' individual characteristics

Variable	Current payers %	Past payers %	Never paid %	All %
Current age				
< 30	15	19	33	20
31–40	51	48	41	48
41–50	32	27	21	28
51+	2	7	5	4
Base	(336)	(122)	(130)	(588)
Chi Sq = 28.12 df = 6; Sig★★★				
Employment status				
employed	74	34	28	54
self-employed	15	9	9	12
inactive	11	57	69	33
Base	(331)	(122)	(129)	(582)
Chi Sq = 178.55 df = 4; Sig★★★				
Highest educational qualification				
no qualifications	26	46	44	34
CSE, GCE, GCSE, School cert	38	31	35	36
ONC/BTECH/A level/higher	15	14	10	14
HNC/Degree/Post Graduates	21	8	10	16
Base	(317)	(111)	(124)	(552)
Chi Sq = 29.99 df = 6; Sig★★★				
Housing tenure				
family/friends and other	13	9	19	14
private owned/mortgage	60	33	21	46
LA/HA and private rent	27	58	60	41
Base	(335)	(122)	(130)	(587)
Chi Sq = 78.92 df = 4; Sig★★★				
Fathers' circumstances now				
very well off	12	6	2	9
comfortably off	22	11	16	18
managing alright	44	46	35	42
not very well off	12	13	20	14
hard pressed	9	25	25	16
Base	(336)	(122)	(130)	(588)
Chi Sq = 45.84 df = 8; Sig★★★				
Savings				
yes, have savings	35	21	17	28
no savings	65	79	83	72
Base	(330)	(122)	(130)	(582)
Chi Sq = 18.90 df = 2; Sig★★★				
Age first became a father				
< 20	8	20	30	15
20–24	37	41	29	36
25–30	38	27	24	33
> 31	17	11	17	16
Base	(333)	(123)	(130)	(586)
Chi Sq = 44.54 df = 6; Sig★★★				

Table 8.1 (cont'd)

Variable	Current payers %	Past payers %	Never paid %	All %
Number of past relationships in which had children				
one past relationship	92	88	82	89
more than one past relationship	7	11	18	11
Base	(336)	(122)	(130)	(588)
Chi Sq = 10.51 df = 2; Sig★★				
Occupation of those employed				
professional/technical/admin	28	23	10	26
clerical/sales/service	20	19	31	22
skilled worker	28	26	28	27
semi–skilled/farm/other	24	32	31	26
Base	(294)	(53)	(39)	(386)
Chi Sq Not Sig				

★p < 0.05; ★★p < 0.01; ★★★p < 0.001.

status of the groups: 74 per cent of current payers were in employment, whereas only 34 per cent of past payers and 28 per cent of never paid fathers were in employment. The picture that emerges from the fathers' individual characteristics is that payers, in comparison to the two groups not paying, were better educated, were economically active, and were more likely to live in owner occupier accommodation, to describe themselves as being financially better off and to have savings. They also seemed to have postponed fatherhood till they were older, and were more likely to have had only one past relationship involving children.

Just under a third of the never paid fathers were under 20 years of age when they first became a father and a third were under 30 years of age at the time of the study. They were the group most likely to have had more than one past partnership involving children – 18 per cent compared with 11 per cent of past payers and only 7 per cent of payers. Their tendency to be younger at the time of the study and their slightly higher multiple past partnership rate could reflect the fact that they were younger when they first became fathers. Additionally, more of the never paid fathers were living with family and friends than in the other two groups, and though financially they were similarly hard pressed to the past payers, fewer of them described themselves as 'managing alright'. Only 35 per cent of the never paid fathers said they were 'managing all right', compared with 44 per cent of current payers and 46 per cent of past payers.

Table 8.2 Payment of maintenance, by former partners' socio-economic circumstances

	Current %	Past %	Never %	All %
Mother lives with new partner				
yes	52	50	42	49
no	41	31	35	37
don't know	8	18	24	13
Base	(335)	(121)	(130)	(586)
Chi Sq = 24.81 df = 4; Sig★★★				
Mother's new partner working				
yes	81	69	52	73
no	9	7	15	9
don't know	10	25	33	18
Base	(173)	(61)	(54)	(288)
Chi Sq = 21.54 df = 4; Sig★★★				
Mother's employment status				
works full-time	32	22	15	26
works part-time	26	14	5	19
not working	17	23	37	22
don't know	25	42	42	32
Base	(334)	(123)	(130)	(587)
Chi Sq = 64.70 df = 6; Sig★★★				
Whether mother on income support				
yes	35	38	44	38
no	36	9	17	25
don't know	29	53	39	37
Base	(228)	(97)	(116)	(441)
Chi Sq = 34.99 df = 4; Sig★★★				
Mother's financial circumstances				
living comfortably	32	23	14	26
doing alright	26	23	23	24
just getting by	21	16	18	19
it's quite/very difficult	9	8	16	10
don't know	12	30	29	19
Base	(327)	(113)	(120)	(559)
Chi sq = 37.23 df = 8; Sig★★★				

★p < 0.05; ★★p < 0.01; ★★★p < 0.001.

Socio-economic circumstances of fathers' last former partner

Though the fathers' socio-economic circumstances were associated with their maintenance status, so too were the socio-economic circumstances of their last former partners, to whom they were paying child maintenance (Table 8.2).

Comparing across the groups, the current payers seemed the best informed about the circumstances of their former partners. Nevertheless the current payers' former partners were also more likely to be living with a new partner, to have partners who were employed, to be working full-time themselves, and to be financially comfortable. Over a third were however said to be in receipt of Income Support. An opposite picture is provided of the circumstances of the former partners of the never paid fathers; nearly half (44 per cent) were known to be in receipt of Income Support and they were more likely to be described as just getting by or finding it quite/very difficult financially.

Though not shown in the table, where the former partners were working or where they were not in receipt of Income Support, they were much more likely to be paid maintenance. Some 69 per cent of those former partners who were known to be working full-time were paid maintenance (and 79 per cent of the part-time workers) compared with only 42 per cent who were not working. Similarly, 74 per cent of the former partners who were not in receipt of Income Support were paid maintenance compared with only 47 per cent who received Income Support.

It seems, therefore, that the potentially poorest mothers – those who were in receipt of Income Support or not working themselves – were the least likely to be paid maintenance.

Fathers' current marital status and household circumstances

Fathers' current family circumstances were also significant factors associated with maintenance payments (Table 8.3).

Though the majority of the fathers in each maintenance group were single, the current payers were most likely to be married or cohabiting with a new partner but not living with children. Even if they were living with children, they tended to have fewer children than the past payers. In addition, where the current payers had new partners, these new partners were most likely to be working full-time – 55 per cent compared with only just over a quarter of the past payers' and only 15 per cent of the never paid fathers' new partners.

These patterns of maintenance payment, by different family and household circumstances, probably reflect both the incomes and the financial demands upon these fathers' households. Thus, it seems the current payers had the most help from the earnings of their current partners, while having fewer demands on their resources from having no children, or fewer children in their households. Though the never paid fathers were the group most likely to be living alone and therefore had the fewest demands on their resources from resident children, they were also most likely to have partners who were economically inactive (like the majority of these fathers of whom over two-thirds were economically inactive).

Fathers' individual characteristics and household arrangements could be described as the more structural elements that may be related to financial ability to pay maintenance. The history of the relationship with former partners and current relations with former partners and children could be described as the 'softer' factors that may be associated with maintenance payment. These are now discussed.

Table 8.3 Payment of maintenance, by fathers' current household arrangements

	Current payers %	*Past payers* %	*Never paid* %	*All* %
Current marital status				
single	54	57	70	58
married	26	29	13	24
cohabiting	20	14	17	18
Base	(336)	(122)	(130)	(588)
Chi Sq = 15.13 df = 4; Sig★★				
Current living arrangements				
lives alone	35	36	40	36
lives with partner only	22	11	8	16
lives with partner and children only	24	33	22	25
lives with parent/other relative	9	7	13	9
other	10	14	16	12
Base	(336)	(122)	(130)	(588)
Chi Sq = 23.67 df = 8; Sig★★				
Number of dependent children in household				
none	74	56	71	70
1	13	25	13	15
2 or more	13	19	15	15
Base	(336)	(122)	(130)	(588)
Chi Sq = 15.57 df = 4; Sig★★				
Father's partner works				
partner works full-time	55	28	15	43
partner works part-time	17	22	12	17
partner inactive	28	50	73	40
Base	(156)	(54)	(41)	(251)
Excludes those partners who were self-employed				
Chi Sq = 38.11 df = 4; Sig★★★				

★p < 0.05; ★★p < 0.01; ★★★p < 0.001.

Table 8.4 Previous history of the relationship with the last former partner, by maintenance status

	Current payers %	Past payers %	Never paid %	All %
Time lived together				
never lived together	8	9	13	9
2 years or less	10	15	25	14
>2 but <5 years	17	19	28	20
>5 but <10 years	27	22	15	24
10 years and over	38	36	19	33
Base	(328)	(115)	(125)	(568)
Chi Sq = 38.06 df = 8; Sig★★★				
Marital status with former partners				
was married, now divorced	64	62	29	55
was married, now separated	12	6	15	11
cohabited but never married	16	23	43	23
never cohabited/never married	8	8	12	9
Base	(335)	(120)	(129)	(584)
Chi Sq = 63.49 df = 6; Sig★★★				
Contact with former partner				
yes, contact	82	59	60	72
no contact	18	41	40	28
Base	(335)	(122)	(130)	(587)
Chi Sq = 43.83 df = 2; Sig★★★				
State of relations with former partners – all fathers				
amicable	63	43	46	55
neither amicable nor hostile	10	9	7	9
hostile – no relationship	27	48	47	36
Base	(332)	(119)	(126)	(577)
Chi Sq = 25.80 df = 4; Sig★★★				

★p < 0.05; ★★p < 0.01; ★★★p < 0.001.

Payment of maintenance, by fathers' relationships with former partners

Table 8.4 demonstrates that among the current and past payers of maintenance, the history of relationships with former partners was very similar; by far the majority in both groups had been married to their former partners and had lived with them for at least five years. The majority of never paid fathers had not been married and had shorter-term relationships. However, it is interesting to note that, although the proportions are small, the never paid fathers were only slightly more likely to have never lived with the mothers of their children compared with current and past payers. This suggests that the majority of their relationships, though shorter generally, were not just fleeting relationships.

The state of current relations with partners provides a slightly different picture. In comparison to current payers, both groups of non-payers (past and never paid fathers) were more likely not to have contact with former partners and to describe their current relations with them as hostile or non-existent. Of course non-payment of maintenance itself may lead to poor relations with former partners and loss of contact. It is therefore impossible to tell in which direction these factors exert influence on one another.

Payment of maintenance, by fathers' relationship with children from last partnership

Compared with the number and ages of the fathers' non-resident children, the most important factor associated with maintenance payment was the fathers' level of contact with their children (Table 8.5). Some 80 per cent of the current payers had shared care or frequent weekly to monthly contact, whereas over a quarter of the past payers, and over a third of the never paid fathers, saw their children less often than once a year if at all.

However, current payers also tended to have both more non-resident children and older non-resident children than the rest. These factors are probably related to the length of the fathers' relationships with the children's mothers. As already highlighted, the majority of current payers had longer-term relationships with mothers, thus the age of their youngest non-resident child would be older, and presumably the longer the parents' relationship, the more chance there would be of having more than one child.

The sex of children and the distance fathers lived from their children's homes (measured in miles) were not significant factors associated with maintenance payment.

Types of maintenance arrangements

Another important factor that may have contributed to whether fathers paid maintenance was the kind of arrangement made. Table 8.6 describes whether fathers ever had, or never had, a formal arrangement in place to pay maintenance through the CSA/courts or DSS. It seems that overall the majority of fathers (54 per cent) never had formal arrangements. But comparing across the groups, the majority of current payers (57 per cent) had made a formal arrangement at some time,

Table 8.5 Payment of maintenance, by numbers of non-resident children and by fathers' relationship with non-resident children from last partnership

	Current payers %	Past payers %	Never paid %	All %
No. of non-resident children				
1	54	62	70	60
2	37	34	22	33
3 and above	8	4	8	7
Base	(336)	(121)	(129)	(586)
Chi Sq = 12.50 df = 4; Sig★★				
Age of youngest child				
0–4 years	16	20	32	20
5–10 years	47	35	47	45
11–18 years	37	44	21	35
Base	(336)	(121)	(129)	(586)
Chi Sq = 25.49 df = 4; Sig★★★				
Contact with children				
shared care	5	7	5	5
weekly to at least once per month	75	53	46	64
once every three months to once or twice per year	8	15	10	10
less often than once per year to never	11	26	38	20
Base	(330)	(121)	(128)	(579)
Chi Sq = 53.68 df = 6; Sig★★★				
Involvement in decisions over children for fathers who have seen child in last year				
about right	42	26	40	38
not often enough	26	20	17	23
never	32	53	42	38
Base	(308)	(97)	(90)	(495)
Chi Sq = 17.15 df = 4; Sig★★				

★$p < 0.05$; ★★$p < 0.01$; ★★★$p < 0.001$.

whereas only a minority of never paid fathers (15 per cent) had made one. This means that only a minority of fathers (3 per cent of the sample as a whole) had actually *never complied* with a legal maintenance arrangement (or at least admitted to it). It was not possible to tell how many of the past payers had defaulted on their legal agreements, as the data reflect all arrangements made over time. Thus, formal agreements made through the courts may not have been in force at the time of the study.

The fact that more of the current payers had formal agreements could be explained in two ways. First, since the majority were already paying maintenance (and were therefore not defaulting on payment) they may have been more willing to admit to having a formal arrangement.

Table 8.6 Whether fathers ever had a formal arrangement to pay
maintenance, by maintenance status

	Current payers %	Past payers %	Never paid %	All %
Ever had formal agreement CSA/Court/DSS	57	50	15	46
No formal agreement	42	51	85	54
Base	(334)	(122)	(128)	(584)
Chi Sq = 68.31 df = 2 Sig★★★				

★★★p < 0.001.

Table 8.7 Type of maintenance arrangement

	Current payers %	Past payers %	Never paid %	All %
Through the courts	34	34	8	28
Through the DSS	4	6	1	4
Through the CSA	21	14	7	16
Informally between parents	40	43	12	35
Father arranged alone	4	13	4	6
Other	4	2	—	2
No arrangements	—	—	72	16
Base	(334)	(123)	(128)	(585)

Multiple responses.

Second, as the majority were ex-married men, the legal proceeding
of divorce would necessarily involve negotiations about maintenance
for children.

A detailed breakdown of all types of arrangements is provided in
Table 8.7. Given that the survey was conducted between April 1995
and April 1996, some two to three years after implementation of the
Child Support Act in April 1993, very few fathers had a Child Support
Agency assessment (16 per cent) and others would not have qualified
for a Child Support Agency assessment. A full discussion on Child
Support Agency assessments follows in Chapter 10.

Variations in the payment of maintenance

As we have seen, there is considerable variation in the proportion of
fathers with different characteristics paying maintenance. The picture

that emerges is that the current payers of maintenance were in better positions financially, being most likely to be employed, to have partners who were working full-time, and to have no children or fewer children in their households making demands on their resources. Additionally they tended to have had longer-term relationships with the mothers of their non-resident children, to have amicable relations with her and frequent contact with their children. However, in order to identify the most salient factors associated with the payment of maintenance we have undertaken logistic regression. Table 8.8 presents the results of an analysis of the factors which have a bearing on whether child support is currently being paid. The table follows the same patterns used in the regressions presented earlier. The best-fitting model shows that maintenance is less likely to be paid if the father is inactive, if he was under 20 when he first became a father, if he does not provide informal support, if he had never made a formal arrangement for paying maintenance, if he had cohabited with the mother, if the mother was in receipt of Income Support and if he had no contact with the mother. Thus the regression shows that contact with the mother overrides contact with children when it comes to paying maintenance. Additionally it may help to explain some of the discrepancy between reports on maintenance from lone mothers (who are mainly dependent on Income Support), and those from a population of non-resident fathers. For where the mothers were not in receipt of Income Support, the odds of them receiving maintenance were increased more than five-fold.

Table 8.8 Factors associated with the chances of currently paying child support, bivariate and multivariate analysis

Variable	Bivariate	Simultaneous	Best-fitting
Net income quintile			
1	1.00	1.00	
2	1.38	0.34	
3	4.24★★★	0.54	
4	15.26★★★	1.60	
5	19.75★★★	1.80	
don't know income	3.61★★★	0.48	
Employment status			
employed	1.00	1.00	1.00
self-employed	0.67	0.79	0.77
inactive	0.06★★★	0.04★★★	0.05★★★
Current marital status			
single	1.00	1.00	
married	1.50★	0.60	
cohabiting	1.58★	1.31	

Table 8.8 (cont'd)

Variable	Bivariate	Simultaneous	Best-fitting
Current family circumstances			
lives with children	1.00	1.00	
no children	2.08★★★	0.55	
lives alone	1.29	0.28	
Age when first became a father			
under 20	1.00	1.00	1.00
20–24	3.29★★★	3.65★★	3.49★★
25–30	4.78★★★	5.61★★	4.00★★
31+	3.76★★★	6.40★★	3.84★
Marital status with mother			
married now divorced	1.00	1.00	1.00
married now separated	0.80	0.90	1.13
cohabited never married	0.33★★★	0.43	0.45★
never lived with mother	0.52★	5.66	2.08
Time lived with mother			
less than 1 year	1.00	1.00	
1–4 years	1.27	5.91	
5–9 years	2.51★★★	3.99	
10 or more years	2.44★★★	1.30	
Time since separation			
less than two years	1.00	1.00	
2–5 years	1.05	0.84	
5–9 years	1.19	0.56	
10 or more years	0.85	0.55	
Distance lived from child			
0–9 miles	1.00	1.00	
10–25 miles	1.27	1.37	
26+ miles	0.77	0.45	
Age of youngest child			
0–4 years	1.00	1.00	
5–10 years	1.95★★	1.74	
11–18 years	1.90★★	2.36	
Number of non-resident children			
one	1.00	1.00	
two	1.62★★	1.49	
three or more	1.77	6.21★	
Contact with child			
no	1.00	1.00	
yes	3.29★★★	1.21	
Mother's employment status			
working	1.00	1.00	
not working	0.27★★★	0.58	
don't know	0.28★★★	0.71	
Mother lives with a new partner			
yes	1.00	1.00	
no	1.10	2.78★	
don't know	0.33★★★	0.55	

Table 8.8 (cont'd)

Variable	Bivariate	Simultaneous	Best-fitting
Mother receives Income Support			
yes	1.00	1.00	1.00
no	3.16★★★	6.69★★★	5.30★★★
don't know	0.76	1.48	1.33
Contact with mother			
yes	1.00	1.00	1.00
no	0.29★★★	0.45	0.36★★
Relations with mother			
amiable	1.00	1.00	
amiable/distant	1.29	2.35	
not amiable	0.72	1.77	
no relationship	0.26★★	1.34	
Gives informal support			
no	1.00	1.00	1.00
yes	4.27★★★	2.35	3.17★★
Maintenance arrangement			
court/DSS/CSA at some time	1.00	1.00	1.00
no formal arrangement	0.33★★★	0.07★★★	0.11★★★
Assessed by the CSA			
yes	1.00	1.00	
no	0.75★	1.11	

Total number of cases in regression = 360.
★p < 0.05; ★★p < 0.01; ★★★p < 0.001.

Reasons for non-payment

So far the analysis has focused on the factors that may influence payment of maintenance, but non-paying fathers were also asked to give an account of why they had either never paid or why they had stopped paying. Their reasons are outlined in Tables 8.9 and 8.10.

Never-paid fathers

The most common reasons given for never having paid maintenance were either unemployment (33 per cent), or not being able to afford maintenance (30 per cent). However, one-quarter gave reasons other than those listed for non-payment. Only a few fathers suggested that they never paid maintenance because they had made either a capital or cash settlement with the mother (10 per cent); or because they did not know where the children and the mother were (9 per cent); or because the father preferred not to pay (6 per cent). Very few said they did not pay because the mother and children did not need it.

Table 8.9 Fathers' reasons for never paying maintenance

	% of cases
Father unemployed	33
Cannot afford to pay	30
Mother prefers not to receive any	18
Mother receives Social Security	15
Mother received family home/lump sum	10
Don't know where children are	9
Father prefers not to pay	6
Shared child-care arrangements	6
Father's current family needs greater	4
Maintenance being arranged	3
Mother and children do not need any	2
Reasons other than above	25
Refused	1
Base	(128)

Percentage of cases giving each response.

Table 8.10 Reasons for stopping paying maintenance for fathers who had paid in the past

	Main reason %	Most popular reason %
Father became unemployed	27	14
Father's finances worsened	10	14
Mother obstructed contact	7	5
Mother remarried/repartnered	6	3
Minimal/no contact with child	5	6
Mother wanted payments to stop	5	3
Mother financially well off	3	3
Amount too high	2	2
Amount was increased	—	—
Father wanted to stop paying	—	2
Mother on Income Support	—	2
Father remarried/repartnered	—	1
Don't know why	—	3
Other**	19	11
No reason/none	11	30
Base: 128 cases		

** reasons not specified.

Some 18 per cent said they never paid because the mother preferred not to receive any maintenance. This finding is comparable to that in Bradshaw and Millar's study where 20 per cent of all lone parents said they did not receive maintenance because they preferred not to have it (Bradshaw and Millar, 1991, Table 7.2: 80).

Past payers

The fathers who had paid in the past also highlighted economic factors for non-payment; 27 per cent said they stopped because they became unemployed, and a further 10 per cent said it was because their financial situation had worsened (see Table 8.10). However, nearly a fifth had other reasons for stopping payments.

Paying potential

We have seen that non-payment of maintenance is related to whether the father is in employment. The question arises: What scope is there for increasing the proportion of fathers who are paying maintenance? If there was to be an effective child support regime, what would be its target? What evidence is there that non-payers are financially able to pay but nevertheless deliberately avoid their obligation? In an attempt to tackle these questions, non-payers were divided into four groups.

Group 1: *No paying potential.* These included the unemployed, non-active, those on Income Support or with equivalent net disposable income in the bottom quintile of the equivalent income distribution and those with shared care of their children[16]. This group consisted of 63 per cent of non-payers. Whether they had paying potential is arguable – the Government proposes to make all fathers pay £5 per week regardless of their circumstances. For those on Income Support with new children this entails distribution from a child in one family to another family who may be better off.

Group 2: *Possible paying potential.* These included those not in Group 1 but who had new family commitments involving children, and equivalent net disposable income in the second and third quintile range, which means that there would be competition for whatever resources were available in the household. They constituted 12 per cent of the non-payers.

Group 3: *Probable paying potential.* These had income in the second and third quintile of the income distribution, but no new family commitments, which meant that there was no competition for household resources. They consisted of 15 per cent of the non-payers.

Group 4: *Certain paying potential.* They were not in the previous three groups and had income in the top two quintiles of the distribution of equivalent income. They consisted of 9 per cent of the non-payers.

These results are summarised in Table 8.11. To check whether the grouping of paying potential had some face validity we looked, as well, at what groups current payers were in. Only 16 per cent of current payers were classified as having no paying potential, whereas 52 per cent of current payers were in the certain paying potential category. Overall these results suggest that there is limited scope for increasing the proportion of non-resident fathers who pay maintenance, though just under a quarter of non-payers had some probable or certain capacity to pay.

Table 8.11 Paying potential

	Current payers %	Non-payers %	All %
Group 1: No paying potential	16	63	38
Group 2: Possible paying potential	14	12	13
Group 3: Probable paying potential	19	15	17
Group 4: Certain paying potential	52	9	32
% of total	54	46	100
Number	226	197	423

In a search for further explanations for non-payment, we examined the non-payers' characteristics. The results are summarised in Table 8.12. Two characteristics were associated with potential to pay maintenance: contact with children and cases where fathers never had a formal maintenance agreement. Non-payers classified as having a certain paying potential were the least likely to have regular contact with their children. They were also the most likely to have never made a formal agreement, though this could reflect that the mother was richer and not on benefit.

In contrast, those with a *probable potential* to pay had the greatest involvement in their children's lives. Some 73 per cent were in regular weekly to monthly contact, and 80 per cent claimed to be giving informal support. It is possible that their greater involvement with children reflects the fact that they had not formed second families (a characteristic of this group). Non-payment of maintenance among this group of relatively well-off fathers may be partly explained by the apparently better-off economic circumstances of mothers. Where the mothers were known to have repartnered, the majority of these partners were in employment (67 per cent). Similarly, nearly a third of these mothers were known to be working themselves, the highest known employment rate across the

Table 8.12 Potential capacity to pay among non-payers (includes never paid and past payers)

	No paying potential %	Possible paying potential %	Probable paying potential %	Certain paying potential %	All %
Contact with child					
regular[a]	56	40	73	33	55
infrequent[b]	15	8	7	17	13
yearly–never[c]	27	52	20	50	31
Base	(122)	(25)	(30)	(18)	(195)
Chi Sq = 25.24 df = 12 Sig★★					
Contact with mother	60	40	63	44	57
Base Not Sig	(125)	(25)	(30)	(18)	(198)
Mother has a new partner	43	56	50	50	46
Base Not Sig	(125)	(25)	(30)	(18)	(198)
Mother's partner employed	52	62	67	56	56
Base Not Sig	(54)	(13)	(15)	(9)	(91)
Mother employed full-time or part-time	23	25	32	29	25
Base Not Sig	(125)	(24)	(31)	(17)	(197)
Mother receives Income Support	48	25	42	20	42
Base Not Sig	(109)	(20)	(24)	(15)	(168)
Gives informal support	66	60	80	50	66
Base Not Sig	(125)	(25)	(30)	(18)	(198)
Never lived with mother	14	8	7	—	11
Base Not Sig	(125)	(24)	(30)	(17)	(196)
Not assessed by CSA	83	64	73	94	80
Base Not Sig	(125)	(25)	(30)	(18)	(198)
Never had formal maintenance arrangement	67	62	61	72	66
Base Chi Sq = 8.06 df = 3 Sig★	(123)	(24)	(31)	(18)	(196)
Total %	63	13	15	9	(198)

a Regular contact, shared care or weekly to monthly.
b Infrequent was three-monthly to yearly.
c Yearly–never = fathers had seen child once in last year or had never seen them.
★p < 0.05; ★★p < 0.01; ★★★p < 0.001.

groups. However, 42 per cent of mothers were also known to be receiving Income Support.

In comparison, the non-payers with second families to support who were categorised as possibly being able to pay were the least involved with their non-resident children. Over half had either seen their children only once in the past year or had never seen them. They were also the group who reported the highest rate of repartnering among the mothers, as over half (56 per cent) had repartnered.

The majority of the poorest fathers, defined here as having no capacity to pay maintenance, did have regular contact with their children, yet two-thirds had never had a formal maintenance arrangement. It seemed that this poorest group of fathers also had the poorest mothers; fewer of the mothers had repartnered and where they had, fewer of these partners were employed. Similarly, fewer of the mothers were employed and more of them were known to be receiving Income Support.

SUMMARY

In this sample 57 per cent of non-resident fathers were currently paying child support. This is a much higher proportion than the 30 per cent reported by samples of lone mothers. Part of the difference is explained by the fact that less than half of the ex-partners of these non-resident fathers were still lone mothers and thus were less likely to be dependant on Income Support (non-resident fathers are more likely to pay child support if the mother is not on Income Support). However, it is also probable that this sample of fathers is biased in favour of those fathers who pay child support. Nonetheless nearly half (48 per cent) of the non-payers defined as having no capacity to pay had former partners who were dependent on Income Support and 57 per cent of those former partners were also lone mothers. Therefore, despite the potential bias in the sample, the evidence still points to the receipt of Income Support among lone mothers as accounting for some of the discrepancy in maintenance payments reported among mothers in other surveys and fathers in this survey. There is also the possibility that mothers on Income Support may not know that maintenance is being paid.

We analysed the characteristics of those currently paying child support using bivariate and logistic regression. Other things being equal, payers were much more likely to be in employment, over 20 when they first became a father, the mother does not receive Income Support, they have contact with the mother, the father also provides informal financial support and they have a formal maintenance arrangement. The main reason given by the fathers who were not paying child support was that the father was unemployed or could not afford to pay and the main reason for past payers stopping paying was that the father had become unemployed.

We evaluated the paying potential of non-payers: nearly two-thirds of non-payers were inactive, on Income Support or living on a low income. Only 9 per cent of non-payers were classified as having 'certain paying potential', but only a third of these had any contact with their child and half saw their child rarely or never. These results suggest that there is little scope for a more effective maintenance regime than the

Child Support Agency increasing the proportion of non-resident fathers who pay child support. It also suggests that there are not large numbers of non-resident fathers financially able to pay but who are deliberately avoiding their obligations.

9 The level of financial support

INTRODUCTION

In the previous chapter we were concerned with finding out who paid maintenance, why some fathers did not pay, and ascertaining the potential capacity of non-payers to make cash payments. In this chapter we focus on the actual amounts paid and how these vary, the factors that might explain variations in amounts of maintenance, and whether fathers were satisfied with the amounts they had to pay. We also examine the reliability of payments. All of these are important considerations, not least for mothers and children who may need to rely on this support, but also for policy makers who are involved in setting realistic maintenance levels. As we shall see, one source of dissatisfaction over maintenance payments was the issue of giving support to children directly (providing clothes, etc.) as a preferred alternative to paying maintenance. In this chapter we explore the interaction of formal and informal child support. Additionally we seek to explain variations in the amounts of regular informal support. Finally we consider those who provide no support at all – those who neither pay maintenance nor give regular informal support.

Variations in the amounts of maintenance

The average amount paid by all those who claimed to be making payments was about £26 per week per child. Figure 9.1 shows the distribution of child support per week per child – 10 per cent of the fathers were paying £5 or less per child per week, over half (53 per cent) were paying in the range £16 to £30 per week per child and 9 per cent were paying over £51 per child per week.

Table 9.1 shows that less was paid on average where fathers were economically inactive, where equivalent net income was lower, where fathers lived in a household with partners and children, where they had

Child support

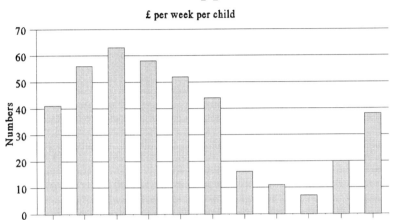

Figure 9.1 Distribution of child support

not made a capital settlement involving the family home, where they did not know whether the mother's former partner was employed, where they lived less than 26 miles away from their children, or where their method of payment was described as 'other'.

It is rather curious that where fathers lived 26 or more miles away from their children they paid more than those who lived closer by. Also if mothers had a working partner, then fathers paid less on average than if the mother's partner was unemployed – £36, compared with £24 if he was employed. This might suggest that employed stepfathers were expected to shoulder some of the financial costs of supporting the non-resident fathers' children. The existence of a capital settlement produced higher maintenance amounts and probably reflects the fact that those who had lived in mortgaged or owned property were better off than those who had rented.

Differences in mean amounts of maintenance were not significantly different by the length of time fathers had lived with mothers, the father's marital status at the birth of the child, the length of time since separation from the mother, the quality of father's relationship with the mother, mother's employment status, whether she received Income Support, whether she lived with a new partner or was a lone parent, or whether the father had made a previous cash settlement. The frequency of contact with non-resident children was also not significant. It is surprising that these factors do not explain variations in mean amounts paid. Some of them were found in Chapter 8 to have an impact on whether maintenance was paid at all. It could be that for those who were paying, the amounts were fixed. They may have been set by the courts and not reviewed or upgraded over time. Certainly there was no significant difference in mean amounts between those who had made a formal agreement at some time (through the courts, DSS or CSA) and those who had never made a formal agreement.

Table 9.1 also presents a summary of the level of total maintenance paid as a proportion of equivalent net disposable income. Overall, 14 per cent of net income was paid in maintenance. Variations in amounts of maintenance as a percentage of net income were only significantly different in respect of employment status and the current household circumstances of the father. Inactive fathers were paying 20 per cent of their net incomes in maintenance and the employed and self-employed 13 and 10 per cent respectively. It seems that the poorest fathers were the most generous in terms of sharing their incomes, even if actual amounts paid were lower for this group than the rest. Where fathers had second families to support, less of their income was spent on maintenance, only 8 per cent by those with a new partner and children compared with 19 per cent by those who were living with others such as relatives or friends.

Table 9.1 Average weekly amount of maintenance per child by current payers and total amount of maintenance paid as a percentage of income

	No.	Mean amount paid £	sd	No.	Mean amount paid as % of income	sd
Employed	234	26.65	19.70	187	13	9.91
Self-employed	48	26.38	28.15	19	10	7.47
Inactive	35	17.03	23.72	25	20	18.27
Total	(316)	25.56	21.75	(232)	14	11.19
F = 3.02 df = 2 Sig★				F = 6.36	Sig★★★	
Quintile net income						
1	21	14.27	18.26	15	16	12.45
2	26	12.38	10.64	26	12	10.49
3	51	21.77	18.61	51	16	16.43
4	69	23.97	16.77	69	14	9.41
5	75	37.16	24.87	75	12	7.42
don't know income	78	25.63	22.81			
Total	(320)	25.53	21.67	(236)	14	11.15
F = 8.65 df = 5 Sig★★★				Not Sig		

Table 9.1 (cont'd)

	No.	Mean amount paid £	sd	No.	Mean amount paid as % of income	sd
Current household						
lives alone	114	25.47	24.36	91	16	11.84
lives with partner only	70	31.31	27.97	42	10	6.51
lives with partner and child only	78	19.42	12.69	56	8	6.12
lives with others	59	28.30	20.02	48	19	13.83
Total	(321)	25.79	22.52	(236)	14	11.15
F = 3.82 df = 3 Sig★★				F = 11.97	Sig★★★	
Capital settlement						
mother kept all	42	31.85	30.11	27	12	7.51
father kept all	17	32.00	33.30	14	9	5.61
value shared	53	31.63	24.64	40	14	8.95
other/not settled yet	62	27.84	20.34	43	13	8.93
no capital settlement	85	19.29	16.28	66	16	15.25
Total	(258)	26.73	23.41	(180)	14	11.36
F = 3.60 df = 4 Sig★★★				Not Sig		
Mother's new partner employed (for those living with a new partner)						
yes	135	23.63	17.01	102	13	11.78
no	15	36.43	35.12	11	12	5.69
don't know	16	14.36	8.74	15	11	8.16
Total	(167)	23.87	19.23	(128)	13	11.02
F = 5.54 df = 2 Sig★★★				Not Sig		
Distance lived from children						
0–9 miles	195	23.38	18.23	148	14	11.86
10–25 miles	53	27.79	22.28	42	13	8.58
26 plus miles	67	33.20	30.95	47	14	11.08
Total	(316)	26.21	22.46	(236)	14	11.15
F = 5.05 df = 2 Sig★★				Not Sig		
Methods of payment						
direct cash/cheque	147	22.56	16.93	112	14	11.31
standing order/direct debit	105	34.46	29.11	76	15	12.21
magistrates court	24	17.35	7.50	18	10	7.79
CSA	32	23.33	22.04	20	15	10.27
other	12	12.91	14.07	10	9	4.20
Total	(321)	25.79	22.52	(236)	14	11.15
F = 7.09 df = 4 Sig★★★				Not Sig		

★p < 0.05; ★★p < 0.01; ★★★p < 0.001.

Multiple regression analysis was undertaken to explain variation in the weekly amounts of maintenance paid per child. Overall, the best-fitting model, summarised in Table 9.2, explained 44 per cent of the variation in maintenance. Not surprisingly, the most important explanatory factor is the employment status of the father. But the age of the father at the birth of his first child was also an important factor – the older the father at the birth of his first child, the more maintenance is paid. Being older when entering first time fatherhood is probably associated with income. Equivalent weekly net income also explains some of the variation in amounts of maintenance. Where fathers have more than one child then the amount of maintenance per child increases. The amount of any cash settlement given slightly increases the amount of maintenance paid. It is likely that the higher the value of cash assets given to mothers at divorce/ separation, then the better off the father, so increasing the amount of maintenance paid. Conversely the longer the father had been separated from the mother, the lower the amount of maintenance paid. This finding did not show up in the individual analysis of variance. Unfortunately it was not possible to include the values of equity foregone on capital settlements as there were too few cases with sufficient information.

Other characteristics of fathers that were tried in the regression but did not explain variations in amounts of maintenance were: father's current marital status, age now, number of dependent children in the father's household, whether the mother was a lone parent or not, time lived with the mother, whether the relationship with the mother was amicable or not and whether the father had debts incurred by the

Table 9.2 Multiple regression analysis of the amount of child support paid per week

Variables	Unstandardised coefficients	Standardised coefficients	Sig
Constant	−30.976		
Employment status	13.84	.172	**
Age when first became a father	1.160	.172	**
Equivalent net household income (HBAIINC)	.045	.454	***
Number of non-resident children	5.683	.134	*
Number of years since separation	−.107	−.147	**
Value of assets given to mother (excluding equity of house)	.0003	.136	**
R square	.44		

*p < 0.05; **p < 0.01; ***p < 0.001.

ending of the relationship. Surprisingly, the existence of a CSA assessment did not explain variations in amounts of maintenance and neither did contact with children. Yet contact with children was associated with whether maintenance was paid or not.

Reliability of maintenance payments

Where fathers were paying maintenance, they were asked about the method used for payment and their reliability in making payments. Table 9.3 shows that only a small minority paid through the courts (7 per cent) or through the CSA (10 per cent). This suggests that the majority were taking responsibility for the transfer of maintenance to former partners, indeed the preferred method of payment was directly to the mother. However, it is hard to say whether those who used banking services had taken responsibility for ensuring that maintenance was paid; some may have had this condition imposed upon them by the court, the DSS or the CSA.

Table 9.3 Types of maintenance by current payers of maintenance

	%
Direct by cash/cheque	46
Standing order/direct debit	33
Through magistrates court	7
Through CSA	10
By other means	4
Base	(334)

There was an association between regularity of payment and whether fathers were currently paying or had paid in the past (Table 9.4). The majority of current payers (88 per cent) said their payments were completely reliable, whereas past payers were more likely to have said that they had missed payments. These findings on reliability among past payers were similar to those in the government's review of court and DSS cases reported in 'Children Come First' in 1990. The review found that two in five DSS cases had one or more periods when the liable parent did not pay (para 5.1.2) and in magistrates cases one in three (who had maintenance orders that had resulted in enforcement action) did not pay at some time (para 5.1.3). The two studies are not directly comparable, as the data in 'Children Come First' came exclusively from parents (both liable mothers and fathers) with court or DSS orders and agreements. Also no evidence was collected from parents with informal maintenance arrangements.

Table 9.4 Reliability of maintenance payments among current payers and past payers

	Current payers %	Past payers %	All %
All the time, no missed payments	88	66	82
Most of the time, occasionally missed payments	9	18	12
Irregularly with frequently missed payments/other	2	15	6
Base	(336)	(122)	(458)
Chi Sq = 39.43 df = 2 Sig★★★			

★★★p < 0.001.

Satisfaction with payments

As well as this high level of perceived reliability in payments among the current payers, most of them (65 per cent) were satisfied with the amount of maintenance they were currently paying. However, 23 per cent were fairly or very dissatisfied with the amount they were paying.

Table 9.5 Levels of satisfaction with amounts of maintenance for current payers

	% of cases
Very satisfied	32
Fairly satisfied	33
Neither satisfied nor dissatisfied	11
Fairly satisfied	9
Very dissatisfied	14
Base	(335)

The very dissatisfied group of paying fathers were asked to give their main reason, second main reason and other reasons for their dissatisfaction. Table 9.6 presents all of these and also ranks the responses in both columns.

The ranking shows that the main reasons for fathers' dissatisfaction were generally economic concerns over the amount to be paid. Over a quarter (26 per cent) said the amount of maintenance was too much, while 13 per cent said the amount over-estimated the cost of bringing up a child. These were ranked first and third respectively in the main reason column. Similarly, the most popular reason for dissatisfaction was

Table 9.6 Reasons for dissatisfaction with amounts of maintenance among fathers who were dissatisfied

	Main reason		Most popular reason	
	Rank	%	Rank	%
Too much money	1	26	1	16
Other reasons	2	17	3	11
Over-estimates cost of child	3	13	5	8
No choice over amount	4	11	2	13
Prefer to spend money directly on child	5	8	2	13
Mother obstructs contact	6	5	7	6
Father gave over family home	7	4	6	7
Father gave lump sum	9	2	8	4
Former family on Income Support so they don't benefit	9	2	8	4
Father needs money more	9	2	6	7
Minimal/no contact with child	9	2	7	6
Father never wanted child	8	3	9	1
Money spent on things that do not benefit the child	8	3	4	9
Don't know	—	—	6	7
Base no. of cases = 78				

where maintenance was too high. However, the rankings in the most popular reason column demonstrate that there was a shift from concerns about issues of affordability towards issues of control over the money. Thus, where fathers said they were dissatisfied with the amount of maintenance, either because they had no control over the amount, or because they preferred to spend the money directly on the children, these increased from being fourth and fifth as the main reason to being the second most popular reason given. Correspondingly dissatisfaction about the money not being spent to benefit the child increased from being ranked eighth as the main reason to being the fourth most popular reason.

Very few fathers said they were dissatisfied with the amount because they had handed over the family home or because they had made a lump sum settlement. Neither did obstruction of contact with children seem a particularly important factor creating dissatisfaction.

Concerns among the dissatisfied fathers in this sample over how the maintenance monies should be spent were not uncommon among other non-resident fathers (see Table 9.7). In the Child Support Agency National Client Satisfaction Surveys for 1992, 1993, 1994 and

Table 9.7 Child Support Agency clients' attitudes to paying maintenance

	1992 %	1993 %	1994 %	1995 %
Someone should only pay maintenance if they can be sure it is spent on the children				
agree	76	79	84	87
disagree	16	11	8	8
don't know	8	—	—	—
It is better to buy the clothes for the children than pay regular maintenance				
agree	26	36	41	37
disagree	51	43	40	47
don't know	23	—	—	—
Base	(265)	(543)	(1,536)	(1,162)

Taken from the National Client Satisfaction Surveys for 1992, 1993, 1994 and 1995.

1995, the vast majority of fathers agreed that people should not pay maintenance unless they can be sure it is spent on the children. A sizeable minority of fathers agreed that it was better to buy clothes for their children than pay maintenance (this is explored further in the qualitative analysis).

Past capital settlements and cash settlements

In Table 9.6 very few fathers said they were dissatisfied with the amount of maintenance paid because of previous cash or capital settlements, yet when the Child Support Act 1991 was implemented fathers complained bitterly that these past financial contributions were not accounted for in maintenance assessments. Eventually pressure led to changes that allowed for the inclusion of past settlements in calculating the amount to be paid. Cash settlements in this sample – defined as money given from insurance/endowment policies, savings/investments, assets/inheritance and pension rights – were uncommon (see Table 9.8). Only about a quarter of all the fathers had made a cash settlement. Current payers were more likely than non-payers to have made a cash settlement. Similarly, just under half of the fathers (47 per cent) who had lived with former partners did not live in owner occupier accommodation and therefore could not make a capital settlement involving the family home (not shown). It seems that complaints in respect of past settlements did not affect as many people as might have been suggested by the outcry at the time, nor did they appear to stop fathers paying maintenance although the amounts they paid may have been less.

Table 9.8 Cash settlements, all fathers

	Current payers %	Past payers %	Never paid %	All %
No cash settlement	67	69	87	72
Yes, cash settlement	33	31	13	28
Base	(335)	(122)	(130)	(587)
Chi Sq = 19.61 df = 2 Sig★★★				

★★★$p < 0.001$.

However, for the fathers who had lived in owner occupier accommodation and where capital settlements had been made, just under a third shared the value with the mother and a further 28 per cent said the mother took all the value of the property (Table 9.9). Although the differences are not statistically significant the ex-partner was more likely to have taken the whole value of the house in cases where fathers were not currently paying child support – suggesting that there may have been a trade-off between child support and capital settlements.

Table 9.9 Capital settlements made by fathers who had lived with former partner in owner occupier accommodation

	Current payers %	Past payers %	Never paid %	All %
Partner took all value	25	39	39	28
Father took all value	10	6	4	9
Value shared	30	33	26	31
Other/not settled	35	22	30	32
Base	(183)	(35)	(23)	(241)

Not significant at the .05 level.

Informal support

Given that the evidence on dissatisfaction over amounts was in part related to issues of control over how the money was spent on children, this may suggest that direct spending on children informally was related to maintenance payments in some way. We were keen to measure all forms of support given by fathers, including informal support such as: presents, clothes, shoes and money given to or saved for children; payment of school fees/trips, holidays, and help with household bills,

Table 9.10 Informal support given by all fathers (excludes shared care)

	Current %	Past %	Never %	All %
Gifts/Xmas/birthday presents	65	20	15	79
Children's clothing (not shoes)	64	21	15	61
Pocket money	67	19	14	57
Children's shoes/boots/sport shoes/trainers	65	20	15	56
Holidays or outings	74	16	10	53
Help with school fees/trips	74	15	10	31
Payments to savings accounts	72	18	10	18
Household or domestic goods	63	16	21	16
Help with other bills	70	14	16	13
Help with housing costs	69	17	13	8
Car expenses	68	16	15	8
Other not specified	56	21	23	6
Mortgage payments	85	6	9	3
None of these	35	31	34	14
Base	(329)	(122)	(97)	(548)

Multiple responses.

goods, mortgage payments and car expenses. As fathers who shared care (where children spend roughly equal amounts of time living with their fathers and their mothers) would by necessity provide some informal support items, they are excluded from this part of the analysis.

Table 9.10 shows that only 14 per cent of the fathers had never given informal support to their children, and that the majority of non-payers were giving some informal support. The most common forms of provision were children's presents, clothes and shoes, children's pocket money and holidays and outings. Very few fathers gave help with general household expenses or housing costs, or car expenses. However, fewer of the non-payers gave informal support, even for the most popular items of children's presents. Of those who said they gave none of the items listed, this was roughly equally split between the three maintenance groups – about a third in each.

Not surprisingly, as some informal support items would be given directly to children, patterns of provision seemed to reflect the amount of contact fathers had with children. Table 9.11 shows that the majority of fathers who had regular weekly to monthly contact with children gave more informal support for all the items listed whereas 79 per cent of those with no contact gave none of the items listed.

Table 9.11 Informal support given by all fathers, by contact with children (excludes shared care)

	Regular %	Infrequent to yearly %	Less than yearly to never %	All %
Gifts/Xmas/birthday presents	79	11	10	78
Children's clothing (not shoes)	85	9	6	59
Pocket money	85	11	4	57
Children's shoes/boots/sport shoes/trainers	85	9	6	54
Holidays or outings	83	11	6	52
Help with school fees/trips	87	11	2	31
Payments to savings accounts	80	11	9	18
Household or domestic goods	87	8	5	15
Help with other bills	84	10	6	13
Help with housing costs	73	18	9	8
Car expenses	77	14	9	7
Other not specified	71	18	10	6
Mortgage payments	79	17	4	3
None of these	10	11	79	15
Base	(350)	(57)	(104)	(511)

Multiple responses.
Regular = weekly to monthly regular contact.
Infrequent = infrequent contact once every three months to once per year.
Never = less frequent contact than once per year to never seen child.

Amounts spent on informal support

The average weekly amounts estimated by the fathers to be spent on informal support for all the respondents was £15.99 per week (Table 9.12). Variations in mean amounts were not significant by whether fathers were currently paying maintenance or not. However, there were significant differences in amounts when expressed as a percentage of the father's equivalent net income. Those who had never paid maintenance were spending double the percentage of their income on informal support compared with current and past payers. So although the never paid fathers were the group least likely to be giving informal support, where they did provide it they spent twice as much of their net incomes as current or past payers (though the numbers were limited).

Nonetheless current payers were also paying maintenance, and thus the total amount spent on financial support (maintenance and informal support) was far greater. The weekly average spent by current payers was £60, representing 21 per cent of their net incomes (Table 9.13). It therefore appears that the past payers were spending the least amount of their net incomes on supporting their children.

Table 9.12 Average weekly amounts of informal support and average amounts expressed as a percentage of income, by maintenance group (excludes shared care)

Group	No. cases	Mean £	sd	No.	Mean %	sd
Current payers	276	17.92	26.52	205	7	10.27
Past payers	87	10.90	23.39	65	6	6.58
Never paid	60	14.55	21.07	41	13	17.40
Base	(423)	15.99	25.30	(311)	8	110.1
Not Sig				F = 5.12	df = 2	Sig★★

★★p < 0.01.

Table 9.13 Average weekly amounts of total support including maintenance and informal support for those who were currently paying maintenance (excludes shared care)

	No. cases	Mean £	sd	No.	Mean %	sd
Current payers	252	60.30	53.05	193	21	17.53

Characteristics of fathers that explain variations in amounts of informal support

Table 9.14 examines variations in fathers' estimates of the value of the informal support they are providing. Informal support was significantly higher where the fathers described themselves as being well off financially, the father was self-employed, the father was previously married but not yet divorced, and where the mother was known to be a lone parent. The highest mean amount was £30.93 per week, given by the previously married but not divorced. Conversely the lowest mean amount was £8.74 per week, spent by those fathers who described themselves as financially hard pressed.

However, when these amounts are expressed as a percentage of net income, then an entirely different picture emerges. Income became a significant factor. The fathers in the bottom income quintile range gave the most informal support when expressed as percentage of net income: 16 per cent. This was a similar proportion of net income given by those who described themselves as financially hard pressed and for those who were economically inactive. Where fathers had two or more children in their households, only 3 per cent of their net incomes was spent

Table 9.14 Average weekly amounts of informal support and as a percentage of net income (excludes shared care)

Group	No. cases	Mean £	sd	No. cases	Mean £	sd
Quintile net income group						
1	51	11.29	14.02	49	16	20.27
2	55	11.53	39.00	58	7	8.46
3	62	10.04	12.40	65	6	7.44
4	62	14.06	18.76	67	5	6.00
5	70	28.13	33.40	73	6	6.61
don't know income	96	38.46	177.7	—	—	—
Base	395	21.10	90.71	311	8	11.01
Not Sig				F = 11.39	Sig★★	
Self-assessed financial status						
very well off	46	24.23	22.61	35	8	9.26
comfortably off	72	20.89	47.06	47	5	5.48
managing alright	191	14.84	20.87	142	6	9.96
not very well off	64	17.49	33.64	49	8	8.66
hard pressed	50	8.74	10.61	37	13	19.64
Base	(423)	16.56	28.69	(311)	7	11.01
F = 2.37 Sig★				F = 3.38	Sig★	
Father's employment status						
employed	245	16.33	20.56	195	5	6.34
self-employed	53	27.46	50.63	21	5	5.91
inactive	123	10.81	14.31	92	13	16.80
Base	(448)	20.21	84.94	(308)	8	11.07
F = 8.19 df = 2 Sig★★★				F = 15.49	Sig★★★	
Marital status with mother						
divorced	254	15.56	27.86	184	6	6.82
married now separated	50	30.93	48.53	29	10	12.61
cohabited/never married	95	13.47	15.24	78	10	14.28
never lived with mother	25	9.87	9.22	20	11	19.97
Base	(424)	16.55	28.66	(311)	7	11.01
F = 5.24 df = 3 Sig★★★				F = 4.23	Sig★★	
Mother repartnered						
yes	213	13.13	16.70	166	6	10.12
no	176	21.70	39.61	118	9	12.21
don't know	34	11.37	13.29	27	9	10.68
Base	(423)	16.55	28.69	(310)	7	11.02
F = 4.99 df = 2 Sig★★				Not Sig		

Table 9.14 (cont'd)

Group	No. cases	Mean £	sd	No. cases	Mean £	sd
Father's household composition						
lives alone	159	16.17	23.98	123	10	13.27
lives with partner only	77	19.11	36.51	46	6	13.23
lives with partner and child only	98	12.02	16.93	71	4	4.12
lives with others	90	19.96	32.27	71	8	8.61
Base	(424)	16.55	28.66	(311)	7	11.01
Not Sig				F = 5.51	Sig★★★	
Children in household						
no children	309	18.45	31.97	224	9	12.39
one child	63	12.58	15.33	49	4	4.80
two children	36	10.95	19.11	27	3	4.74
three+ children	16	8.40	9.64	11	3	3.09
Base	(424)	16.55	28.66	(311)	7	11.01
Not Sig				F = 4.39	Sig★★	

★$p < 0.05$; ★★$p < 0.01$; ★★★$p < 0.001$.

on informal support, probably reflecting the higher demands on their resources from second families. Divorced fathers spent the lowest proportion of their net incomes on informal support, 6 per cent, and the never lived together fathers the most, 11 per cent.

Factors that were not associated with statistically significant variations in informal support were: whether fathers had a CSA assessment, the length of time since fathers had separated from mothers, the length of time fathers had lived with mothers, the quality of relations with mothers, and whether mothers were employed. Surprisingly, variations in mean amounts, or variations as a percentage of net income, were not explained by the frequency of contact fathers had with their children (excluding shared care cases). One might have expected that the greater the frequency of contact with children, the more fathers would spend on informal support, both in cash terms and as a percentage of net income.

The questions that arise from this analysis of informal support are: are the non-payers substituting informal support for maintenance, and what is the capacity of these providers of informal support to pay maintenance? Capacity to pay was defined in the same way as described in Chapter 8.

Average amounts of informal support for non-payers whose capacity to pay maintenance was assessed

The average amounts of weekly informal support for those non-payers of child maintenance providing informal support are presented in Table 9.15 (excluding those who share care). The average amounts are also expressed as a percentage of income. Variations in average amounts across the four groups were significant; those who had the greatest capacity to pay maintenance paid the highest mean amount of informal support. This suggests that although these fathers were not paying maintenance, there was some substitution through informal support payments, though the numbers were small for this category. Even the fathers assessed as having no potential to pay formal child support seemed to be contributing to their children's upkeep, spending nearly £9.00 a week on average. There was no significant difference between the groups in the proportion of income spent on informal support.

Table 9.15 Average weekly amounts of informal support given by non-payers, by their potential capacity to pay maintenance and expressed as a percentage of income (excludes shared care)

Group	No.	Mean £	sd	No.	Mean %	sd
No paying potential	81	8.99	11.75	67	12	16.03
Possible paying potential	15	9.21	9.20	15	5	6.26
Probable paying potential	21	10.59	13.92	21	9	12.16
Certain paying potential	9	25.46	25.54	9	4	2.74
Total	125	10.49	13.78	112	10	13.94
F = 4.27 df = 3 Sig**				Not Sig		

**$p < 0.01$.

Logistic regression of the odds of paying something, either formal maintenance or informal support

The majority of fathers in this study claimed to be giving informal support even if they were not paying maintenance. We therefore carried out a logistic regression of the odds of paying some financial support, whether maintenance or informal support (Table 9.16). The best model identified six factors that affect the likelihood of giving some kind of financial support. Fathers are less likely to give any financial

Table 9.16 Logistic regression on giving some financial support maintenance or informal support

Variable	Bivariate	Simultaneous	Best Fitting
Net income quintile			
1	1.00	1.00	
2	1.18	2.07	
3	2.63★★	1.49	
4 and 5	4.86★★★	6.04	
don't know income	1.77★	4.04	
Employment status			
employed	1.00	1.00	1.00
inactive	0.21★★★	0.28★	0.28★★★
Current marital status			
single	1.00	1.00	
married	0.73	0.89	
cohabiting	1.04	2.91	
Current family circumstances			
lives with children	1.00	1.00	
no children	2.09★★	1.25	
lives alone	1.82★	3.86	
Age when first became a father			
under 20	1.00	1.00	
20–24	2.91★★★	4.09★	
25–30	5.94★★★	5.77★★	
31+	3.76★★★	1.70	
Marital status with mother			
married now divorced/separated	1.00	1.00	
cohabited never married	0.49★★	2.39	
never lived with mother	0.42★★	22.84★	
Time lived with mother			
less than one year	1.00	1.00	
1–4 years	1.27	8.95★	
5–9 years	2.39★★	6.21	
10 or more years	3.76★★★	3.69	
Time since separation			
less than two years	1.00	1.00	
2–5 years	1.15	1.13	
5–9 years	1.30	2.67	
10 or more years	0.50★	0.60	
Distance lived from child			
0–9 miles	1.00	1.00	
10–25 miles	0.82	4.38★	
26+ miles	0.36★★★	1.14	
Age of youngest child			
0–4 years	1.00	1.00	
5–10 years	0.71	0.40	
11–18 years	0.87	1.52	

Table 9.16 (cont'd)

Variable	Bivariate	Simultaneous	Best Fitting
Number of non-resident children			
one	1.00	1.00	1.00
two or more	2.13**	6.34**	2.42*
Contact with child			
no	1.00	1.00	1.00
yes	13.00***	13.68***	4.61***
Mother's employment status			
working	1.00	1.00	
not working	0.21***	1.77	
don't know	0.43**	4.76*	
Mother receives Income Support			
yes	1.00	1.00	1.00
no	0.91	1.41	0.83
don't know	0.23***	0.59	0.31**
Contact with mother			
yes	1.00	1.00	1.00
no	0.08***	0.08***	0.20***
Relations with mother			
amiable/distant	1.00	1.00	
not amiable	0.56	6.16**	
no relationship	0.08***	2.15	
Maintenance arrangement			
court/DSS/CSA at some time	1.00	1.00	1.00
no formal arrangement	0.40***	0.17***	0.27***
Assessed by the CSA			
no	1.00	1.00	
yes	1.62	0.82	

Total number of cases in regression = 361.
*p < 0.05; **p < 0.01; ***p < 0.001.

support if they are inactive, have only one non-resident child, have no contact with the child, have no contact with mother and if they have never had a formal maintenance arrangement. The number of non-resident children is probably masking the effect of marital status/length of living-together relationship. The finding that fathers are no less likely to give some financial support if the mother is on Income Support (it is only significant if fathers do not know whether she is on Income Support) is curious.

SUMMARY

The analysis suggests that current payers on average paid £26 maintenance per child per week. The level of maintenance paid was higher where fathers were employed, they had higher incomes, they were older when they first became a father, they had more than one non-resident child, and where they had given a cash settlement at the time of divorce/separation. The longer the length of time since divorce/separation, the lower the amount paid.

The majority paid their child support directly to their former partners and 88 per cent of current payers said that they paid their child support regularly. Two-thirds of the fathers were satisfied with the amount of maintenance that they paid. Those who were dissatisfied mostly felt that the amounts were too high. A quarter of the fathers had made a previous cash settlement, but they were also more likely to be current payers of child maintenance.

The majority of current payers also gave informal support. Fathers estimated that the average value of informal support was £16 per week. Two-thirds of the never paid fathers claimed to give informal support and of those who provided an estimate, they spent a larger percentage of their income in this way than either the past payers or current payers. Actual amounts spent on informal support also reflected the financial circumstances of fathers. Amounts were greater on average where the father was employed and where he had a higher income and where he described himself as not being 'hard pressed' financially. However, the fathers who were economically inactive or whose incomes were in the lowest quintile range or who described themselves as hard pressed spent the highest proportion of their incomes on informal support compared with the others.

Fathers are less likely to give either formal or informal support if they are inactive, have only one non-resident child, have no contact with the child or mother and if they have no formal maintenance arrangement. In the next chapter we go on to consider what part the Child Support Agency plays in the lives of these men.

10 The Child Support Agency

INTRODUCTION

The Child Support Agency began operations in April 1993 and our survey was in the field between April 1995 and August 1996. We had expected that we would be able to contribute to a preliminary evaluation of how it was operating and what it was achieving. However, there were delays in the take-on of cases for the Child Support Agency and it was decided to focus on cases of lone mothers already in receipt of Income Support and Family Credit and new cases of claims for Income Support. The operation of the Agency changed over the period of the fieldwork, as well as subsequently, not least as a result of new regulations in 1994 and a new Act in 1995 that had the effect of substantially changing the formula. This study is therefore not a particularly good vehicle for exploring the operation of the child support scheme as it is now. Nevertheless, it was considered worthwhile reviewing the fathers' experiences even though it might represent a picture that may have been overtaken by events. In the first part of the chapter we draw on the sample survey and in the second part on the qualitative study of financial support.

QUANTITATIVE SURVEY FINDINGS

Contact with the Child Support Agency

Tables 10.1 and 10.2 present details on contact with the CSA by whether fathers were currently paying maintenance, had done so in the past, or had never paid. The majority of the fathers in the sample had no contact at all with the CSA (57 per cent). Overall, of those who had contact, the past payers were the most likely to have contact with the CSA and the never paid the least likely to have contact. Given that the

Table 10.1 Maintenance group, by contact with the CSA

	Current payers %	Past payers %	Never paid %	All %
Yes, contact with CSA	46	52	27	43
No contact with CSA	54	47	73	57
Base	(335)	(122)	(129)	(586)
Chi Sq = 19.01 df = 2 Sig★★★				

★★★p < 0.001.

Table 10.2 Whether fathers split pre/post April 1993 and whether they had contact with the CSA, by maintenance group

	Split pre 1993 %	Split post 1993 %
Current payers		
Yes, contact with CSA	47	44
No contact with CSA	53	56
Base	(226)	(109)
Past payers		
Yes, contact with CSA	51	56
No contact with CSA	49	44
Base	(88)	(34)
Never paid		
Yes, contact with CSA	23	31
No contact with CSA	76	69
Base	(68)	(61)
Chi Sq = 20.41 df = 5 Sig★★		

★★p < 0.01.

never paid group reported the highest proportion of mothers in receipt of Income Support, some 44 per cent (see Table 8.2 earlier), this supports early criticisms made of the CSA, that they were prioritising 'soft targets'. That is, they were contacting those fathers who had been paying maintenance as opposed to pursuing the so-called 'feckless fathers' who had never paid maintenance (House of Commons, HC 983, 1993). However, contact with the CSA was slightly higher for the never paid fathers if they had separated from former partners following implementation of the Act in April 1993, compared with those who had separated prior to April 1993. Even so, only just under a third of the never paid fathers who separated after implementation of the Act admitted to having any contact with the CSA.

Nature and outcome of contact with CSA

Where contact with the CSA had taken place, this was overwhelmingly initiated by the CSA rather than by the fathers themselves (Table 10.3). The majority who had contact received a Maintenance Enquiry Form (MEF), some 88 per cent, and of those 86 per cent had completed and returned the MEF to the Agency. However, a quarter of the never paid fathers had not returned their MEF, compared with only 13 per cent of current payers and only 10 per cent of past payers. Where the MEFs were not returned (30 cases in total), just over half said it was because they did not want to return it, and just under a quarter did not specify a reason. Hardly anyone said it was because they did not have enough

Table 10.3 Nature of contact with the CSA and the outcome of contact, by fathers' maintenance group

	Current payers %	Past payers %	Never paid %	All %
Respondent contacted CSA first	9	3	17	9
CSA contacted respondent first	91	97	83	91
Base	(155)	(64)	(35)	(254)
Chi Sq = 5.68 df = 2 Sig★				
CSA sent MEF	90	89	80	88
CSA did not send MEF	8	9	14	9
Don't know if MEF sent	2	2	6	2
Base	(155)	(63)	(35)	(253)
Not Sig				
Returned completed MEF	87	89	74	86
Did not return MEF	13	10	26	14
Base	(139)	(57)	(27)	(223)
Not Sig				
Why did not return MEF				
didn't want to return it	39	(4)	(5)	53
not enough information to complete	(1)	—	—	3
advised not to return it	(1)	(1)	(1)	10
still completing it	(2)	—	—	7
didn't know how to fill it in	(1)	—	—	3
other reason	33	—	(1)	23
Base (too few cases to test association)	(18)	(5)	(7)	(30)
CSA sent final/interim assessment	59	56	32	55
No CSA assessment received	41	42	68	45
Base	(150)	(62)	(31)	(243)
Chi Sq = 7.67 df = 2 Sig★				

★p < 0.05; ★★p < 0.01; ★★★p < 0.001.

information to complete it, or that they could not fill in the form. It seems unlikely that fathers were advised by CSA campaign groups not to complete forms, as only 5 per cent were members of any campaign groups.

Though the majority of fathers who had contact with the CSA had both received and returned a MEF, only 55 per cent had received a maintenance assessment at the time of the survey. Comparing across the groups, it was the never paid fathers who were least likely to have received an assessment (68 per cent). There was no statistically significant difference in the proportion of the fathers who had separated before or after the CSA began operating in April 1993 who had received an assessment.

Changes in maintenance amounts

Much has been made of the increases in maintenance amounts brought about by the formula used by the CSA. Indeed, increasing the amounts of maintenance paid was one of the primary objectives of the CSA, though the average amount has since dropped as a result of changes. Nevertheless, one incentive used to encourage compliance is the Interim Maintenance Assessment (IMA). This sets maintenance at an artificially high level and is applied where fathers fail to return the MEF or where information is incomplete. The other type of assessment, the 'Final Maintenance Assessment' (FMA), calculates the amount to be paid based on complete information on fathers' income and expenditures. It should therefore be for a lower amount than the punitively designed IMA.

Given that the majority of the fathers in this sample had completed and returned their MEF, only 13 per cent of those who had received an assessment had an IMA at the time of the study (see Table 10.4). The average weekly amounts of maintenance for those with an IMA did appear

Table 10.4 Change in amount of maintenance, by type of CSA assessment for fathers who had received a CSA assessment

	Final assessment %	Interim assessment %	All %
Gone up	41	33	40
Stayed the same	31	53	34
Gone down	29	13	26
Base	(98)	(15)	(113)

Too few cases to test for association.

Table 10.5 Weekly amounts of CSA maintenance and amount of CSA maintenance as a percentage of net income for all fathers with CSA assessments

	No.	Mean £	sd	No.	Mean %	sd
Final assessment	83	48.64	38.00	81	19	29.73
Interim assessment	12	91.19	34.67	26	25	55.22

Not sig at the .05 level.

Table 10.6 Started payments, by different type of CSA assessment

	Final assessment %	Interim assessment %	All %
Yes, started paying	66	27	61
Not started paying	34	73	39
Base	(100)	(15)	(115)
Chi Sq = 8.47 df = 1 Sig★★			

★★p < 0.01.

to be higher than the FMAs − £91.19 per week on average compared with £48.64 per week for those with FMAs. Similarly, as a percentage of net income, interim assessments were higher, making up 25 per cent of net income (Table 10.5). Final assessments made up 19 per cent of net income. These differences, however, were not significant.

Although the IMAs appeared higher on average, only one-third with IMAs said that their maintenance had been increased, while 13 per cent said the amount had actually been decreased (Table 10.4). Among those with an FMA, 29 per cent had had the amount decreased and more, 41 per cent, had the amount increased (Table 10.4).

Obviously where the IMA assessment had decreased the amount fathers were previously expected to pay − or for the 53 per cent of fathers with an IMA whose amounts had stayed the same − there was little incentive to co-operate with the CSA. Indeed nearly three-quarters of all the IMAs were not being paid regardless of whether the amount was changed (see Table 10.6). Although the numbers of cases here are very small, this finding concurs with the CSA's own figures; of those with IMAs in November 1997 some 90 per cent were not paying any of it (DSS, 1998: 35). However, given that this assessment is applied where there is incomplete information, this may reflect those cases that are still awaiting a Final Maintenance Assessment. Nonetheless over a third with FMAs in this study were not paying this assessment. This is a slightly higher non-compliance rate than found among all the CSA clients, 30 per cent of whom were not paying their FMA in November 1997 (DSS, 1998: 35).

Although 39 per cent of all the fathers who had received an assessment had not started to pay it, this does not mean to say they were not paying any maintenance, only that they had not begun to pay what was required from the CSA. There was a small group of fathers who were not paying their CSA assessment but who still claimed to be paying maintenance − 21 cases representing 16 per cent of all those with a CSA assessment. This small group of fathers paid on average £35.78 per week (Table 10.7). This was less than those fathers who had no CSA assessment but were paying maintenance; they paid £41.41 per week on average. It was also less on average than the amounts paid by those who were paying their CSA assessment; they paid £47.04 per week. However, these apparent differences in mean amounts and as a percentage of income were not statistically significant.

Table 10.7 Average weekly amounts of maintenance paid, by whether paying or not paying CSA assessment and amounts expressed as a percentage of net income

	No.	Mean £ per week	sd	No.	Mean % of net income	sd
Payers paying CSA assessment	54	47.04	30.78	44	15	9.41
Payers with CSA assessment but not paying it	21	35.78	57.53	12	13	7.79
Payers with no CSA assessment	179	41.41	41.82	173	13	11.79

Not sig at the .05 level.

Fairness of CSA assessment

In order to understand why fathers may not have been paying the CSA assessment, they were asked whether they felt that the amount set by the CSA was fair or unfair (Table 10.8). As might be expected, the majority of fathers with an increased assessment felt it was unfair (77 per cent), but so did the majority of fathers who had a decreased assessment (57 per cent), while the majority whose assessment had remained the same thought it was fair. It could be that any change by the CSA was considered unfair, or the results may simply reflect the small numbers of cases.

Table 10.8 Fairness of assessments for all fathers who had a CSA assessment

	Up[a] %	Down[a] %	Same[a] %	All %
Unfair assessment	77	57	43	61
Fair assessment	22	43	57	39
Base	(40)	(28)	(30)	(98)
Chi Sq = 8.705 df = 2 Sig★★				

a = Where CSA had increased, decreased or kept the amount of maintenance the same as previous arrangements.
★★p < 0.01.

Table 10.9 Reasons given for feeling that the amount set by the CSA was unfair, by whether CSA assessment increased, decreased or kept the amount to be paid the same

	Up %	Down %	Same %	All %
Not enough account of living expenses	95	61	72	81
No account of work travel costs	38	56	43	44
Not enough account of housing costs	68	58	48	61
No account of costs of seeing children	53	33	73	53
Not enough account of fathers' current family needs	44	33	28	37
Previously made clean break/lump sum settlement	25	15	35	25
Leave father much worse off	71	49	48	60
Children on IS so don't benefit	33	24	38	32
No account of debts	60	38	46	50
Amount too high	85	52	67	72
Other	8	9	14	10
Base	(35)	(18)	(18)	(70)

Multiple response so % refers to cases giving each response.

Those who thought it unfair were also asked why that was the case. Table 10.9 sets out the answers to these questions by whether the CSA increased, decreased or kept the amount the same. The most popular reasons given were: that it did not take enough account of living expenses (81 per cent), that the amount was felt to be too high (72 per cent), that it did not take enough account of housing costs (61 per cent), that it left the father much worse off financially (60 per cent), that it did not take account of costs of seeing children (53 per cent) and that it did not take account of debts (50 per cent). But a majority of fathers whose maintenance had either stayed the same or had decreased also felt that the amount set by the agency was too high and that it did not take enough account of living expenses. This could mean that these fathers also regarded their previous maintenance arrangements in the same way and therefore it is difficult to say whether this sense of unfairness was related to the CSA specifically, especially given the small number of cases.

Potential behavioural impact of CSA assessments

Table 10.10 describes the impact of CSA assessments on fathers' and/or their partners' behaviour (if they had a partner) by whether their maintenance assessment was increased, decreased or stayed the same.

The group whose behaviour seemed to be affected the most were the fathers whose maintenance had been increased following the CSA assessment. Only 16 per cent said their behaviour would not be affected in any of the ways described, with just under half saying their informal support to children would be affected. One in three also said they would be put off becoming a father again, and about one in four said

Table 10.10 Potential impact of CSA assessment on fathers' or their current partners' behaviour, by whether their maintenance was increased, decreased or not changed following CSA assessment

Q. *Do you think that the CSA assessment has made or will make you (or your current partner) do any of these things?*

	Up %	Down %	Same %	All %
Work fewer hours	24	6	16	17
Give up work	27	35	15	25
Take extra work	16	13	10	13
Change jobs to reduce travel-to-work time	—	4	5	3
Take a second job	2	10	5	5
Partner take paid work	7	9	3	6
Not seek promotion	8	14	7	9
Seek residency of children	13	13	5	10
Seek other contact with children	11	2	4	6
Stop/reduce informal monies/gifts for children	48	22	21	32
Put you off becoming a father again	33	36	22	30
Put you off having another partner	19	25	21	21
None of these	16	32	54	33
Base	(44)	(30)	(38)	(113)

the CSA assessment would make them or their partner work fewer hours or give up work altogether.

Rather incongruously, more of the fathers whose maintenance had been decreased said they or their partner would give up work. This could be a feature of the limited numbers in this part of the analysis or it could be that these fathers anticipate a future rise in their maintenance assessment, which would cause them or their partner to give up work. Findings from the qualitative study on financial obligations help cast further light on the attitudes and behaviour of fathers in regard to the impact of the CSA.

FINDINGS FROM THE QUALITATIVE STUDY ON THE CHILD SUPPORT AGENCY

The fairness of maintenance amounts

All of the eighteen fathers in the second qualitative study that examined financial obligations expressed general concerns about the 'economic fairness' of assessments made by the CSA. These were: fathers should pay only if they could 'afford to', they should have enough money left over for their own current needs and future needs to build a new family, they should have enough money left over for their second families, no account should be taken of the earnings of fathers' partners, some account should be taken of stepfathers' earnings, and they should not have to pay if the mother's earnings were higher than the father's. Overall it was felt to be unfair if the CSA failed to pay heed to these conditions.

Though these fathers expressed general concerns about economic fairness, these were, in most cases, informed by stories picked up in the media, particularly the reporting of suicides following increases of maintenance by the CSA. Of the eighteen respondents, only three were paying CSA assessments and of those only one was employed and was currently experiencing the effects of having his maintenance increased. The two who were unemployed were paying the minimal amount set by the CSA (reported as £5 per week) and this maintenance was deducted at source from their Income Support. Two other fathers were being assessed at the time of interview.

Though only one father had actually experienced an increase in his maintenance following CSA involvement, his case provides some interesting insights into the behavioural consequences resulting from paying a higher amount of maintenance.

Some consequences of increasing maintenance amounts

Peter's (pseudonym) increased maintenance liability following the CSA assessment had an impact in two interrelated ways. First, the higher amounts of maintenance meant he gave less in informal support for his three children. Second, this reduction in informal support led to subtle changes in everybody's behaviour.

According to Peter, while paying maintenance, he also took the major responsibility for providing clothing and shoes for his children, an arrangement he claimed was agreed with the mother. However, when the CSA increased his maintenance by £40 a month he could no longer afford to carry on with this arrangement. This in turn affected the mother's behaviour; she now resorted to emotional blackmail to persuade Peter to buy shoes. Peter described the situation thus:

> That's why, I got a bit annoyed at the beginning; cause you pay £120 to the CSA and then a few days later you'd get a call [phone call from mother] . . . em '[name of oldest daughter] hasn't got any shoes and if you don't get her any shoes then I'll send her to school in her slippers', and you can't send kids to school in slippers so I'd go out and buy them a pair of shoes. But I weren't happy about it cause I'd just spent £120, and now I were having to spend another £20.

However, the difficulty of affordability was exacerbated because of Peter's parental rule of treating all his children equally. Thus:

> But once I'd bought one of them a pair of shoes, so I had to buy another pair of shoes and another pair of shoes for the third one. So your £20 soon became £60 and it got silly, I were skint all the time and I hadn't any money spare to do what I wanted to do. So I weren't too happy at that point. I blame the CSA more than do [ex-wife], because we had it settled before the CSA got involved, we were fine before the CSA got involved.

Peter said 'everybody suffered' as a consequence of CSA involvement. His children no longer received the same amount of new clothes and shoes and they could no longer go on holiday with their father or be treated to days out. Peter despaired because of his inability to provide in this way and he felt his emotional relationship with his children had deteriorated as a result. Indeed, the very core of Peter's fathering was made manifest through the provision of informal support, as it was apparent that this was the main means through which he expressed his love and commitment 'to' his children. The evidence for this lay in his explanation of his own upbringing as a child.

Peter was brought up by his stepfather and he described how, when anything was being bought, he was 'pushed to the back of the queue' behind his stepfather's natural children. This experience had profoundly affected him and he explained:

> there was no way my children would have to go through what I had been through.

This commitment to his children was expressed through his provision of informal support and not through maintenance payments. Giving informal support was an important aspect of his emotional relationship with his children, both in a direct sense, when he treated them to days out, but also indirectly when he wanted to make sure that his children's needs for clothes and shoes were being met. Peter knew that this kind of informal support was a vital contribution to their well-being as their mother (and her husband) were unemployed and dependent on Income Support. Often they could not afford to buy the children what they needed and it was the mother's poverty and resultant dependency on Income Support that was at the root of Peter's problem.

Following involvement of the CSA, the mother's overall income was reduced. She no longer received any of the maintenance paid by Peter, as all of it was clawed back from her Income Support. Consequently Peter felt that the maintenance money was now used for general household expenses to support the mother's husband and their new child, rather than being used specifically for the benefit of his children. As a result, Peter began to object to paying maintenance and at one point he stopped paying, having previously been reliable. From Peter's perspective he felt that he was now the main breadwinner for the mother's household and he was adamant that that responsibility belonged to the mother's new husband. Peter therefore concluded that the CSA's involvement made 'everybody' unhappy.

On the surface this unhappiness was directly related to the financial and emotional consequences of paying more in maintenance and less in informal support. But at a deeper level this unhappiness was related to behavioural changes. According to Peter, the children had become very resentful of their mother because she could not make up the loss of informal support. The mother could not provide adequate clothing or take them swimming or for days out. This resentment expressed itself in the children's behaviour, presenting both parents with difficulties in disciplining the children across two households. In particular, Peter felt torn between supporting the mother in disciplining the children (something he said he had always done) or sympathising with the children in their resentment against the mother. As a result, Peter became highly critical of the mother and her husband, disparaging their dependency on Income Support. He no longer accepted that the husband could not find paid work, having previously been sympathetic. In Peter's eyes even a job 'cleaning public toilets' was a work option that the husband should consider. The increases in maintenance and the overlap between the benefit system and the child support system served to create tensions in cross-household relations, which apparently were either non-existent, or minimal, prior to CSA involvement.

Peter's commitment to providing financial support for his children seemed strong. However, the effect of CSA involvement made him much more ambivalent about the legal obligation to pay maintenance under this system. This ambivalence found expression in his temporary withdrawal of maintenance.

Certainly the issue of financial fairness surrounding the amounts of maintenance set by the CSA is an important concern for fathers, particularly when no amount of maintenance is disregarded in assessing Income Support. In such cases none of the maintenance paid by fathers increases the mother's household income, despite fathers paying more in maintenance. Peter's case clearly demonstrates how the lack of a maintenance disregard serves only to redistribute poverty across the mother's and father's households. Ultimately it is the children who suffer and if Peter's case is in any way typical, then the suffering is both material and emotional as cross-household family relations are put under additional strain.

However, to focus only on those fathers who had CSA assessments would miss the hidden behaviour of some of the other fathers in the qualitative study. There were another four fathers who had previous contact with the CSA but had managed to avoid being assessed. Their behavioural responses to the CSA are also worth exploring in some detail.

Avoiding the CSA

Of the four who had avoided assessments, two, Rhidian and Alex (pseudonyms), could be deemed untypical cases. Rhidian had two non-resident children from his failed marriage. Over the years the children had remained resident with the mother and Rhidian had contact with them every weekend. However, when his son reached 14 years of age he came to live with his father. This change in residency also altered the status of the parents; both were now simultaneously parents with care and absent parents (in CSA terminology); it was at this point that the CSA became involved. In principle, each parent owed the other maintenance and this was problematic as the father was not working (he was a student) yet the mother was. She would therefore have carried the burden of maintenance payments. To avoid this liability the mother gave up her full-time job and began working part-time, and although Rhidian was not entirely clear about how this halted further involvement by the CSA, nonetheless according to Rhidian it did. Neither parent was assessed by the CSA and neither parent paid any maintenance to the other. According to Rhidian they were both satisfied with this arrangement.

Alex had one non-resident child from a cohabiting relationship that had lasted for four years. This child was now 6 years of age and Alex had no contact since the relationship ended, the child being 6 months old at the time. He also never paid maintenance. Contact had not been successfully established because the mother told Alex that he was not the biological father; indeed this was the cause of relationship breakdown. Despite this denial of his paternity, Alex remained doubtful about his biological status and he tried, with the aid of his solicitor, to remain in contact with the child following separation, but with no success. He described his feelings thus:

> I was only with her [the child] for the first 6 months anyway, and then I was told that I wasn't the father of the baby, then I was told there wasn't any need to see her. So it was just like something being taken away from you, it was hard. Because obviously the first six months of her life I actually thought she was my daughter and then all of a sudden she wasn't, it was just like being kicked in the teeth if you want to put it that way, it was hard.

Over the years he had come to believe that he was not the actual father, otherwise he said the mother would have at least kept him informed about the child's well-being. However, the possibility that he was the father preyed on his mind, especially as Alex was adopted himself and he had always wanted to know his own biological parents. Consequently, as it seemed the mother was naming him as the father to the CSA (the child still carried Alex's surname) but not to Alex, he was now very perturbed about what his responsibilities to this child should be. Alex was adamant that he wanted a DNA test to clarify his biological relationship – yet despite this he made no plans to have a paternity test. The CSA's involvement had forced him to revisit both the doubts over his paternity and the pain over the loss of this child; his anger at the mother was still very apparent at the time of interview.

> You've got to remember I was in a relationship prior to her having the baby, I was treating her as somebody I loved and somebody I wanted to marry, then all of a sudden she turns round, this person who loves you and says 'You're not the father of my baby' so what am I going to think? You cannot actually put down in words what I would like to say.

Alex was incensed about the intrusion of the CSA into his life and although he was not explicit about how he avoided being assessed, he did suggest that he had managed to sidestep the Agency.

Both of these cases demonstrate the difficulties posed in defining 'non-resident fatherhood' within a rigid administrative system such as the CSA. First, before any liability for maintenance can be assessed, the biological status of the father has to be proved in some cases. Though the Agency has the means to determine paternity, it is hard to imagine the effects on men (and women and children) of proving this paternity retrospectively, especially when all parties had long ago learned to accept such ambiguities. Other fathers may not even know of the existence of a child until the Agency becomes involved. If the scientific advances in DNA testing were not available, the Agency would be more reliant on the parents' own acknowledgement of the existence of a meaningful relationship between fathers and children. Less primacy would necessarily be placed upon 'biological' obligations alone, as opposed to a combination of 'biological and social' obligations. The difficulty posed for Alex by the CSA's involvement was to assimilate his past feelings for this child, while simultaneously deciding about his future responsibilities to this child – if paternity was proved. Being forced to connect past and future feelings/responsibilities in this way was not something Alex relished and he sought comfort by trying to ignore the possibility that he was the father, hence his reluctance to pursue DNA testing. After all, from Alex's viewpoint the mother had made it clear that she did not want him in the child's life.

Second, the degree of 'absence' of one parent has to be defined for maintenance purposes and this may change over time. To continually define 'absence' or 'non-residence' presents the Agency with a difficult task, as it must follow the private movements and emotional allegiances of children across their parents' households. It is therefore debatable if

Rhidian and the mother were colluding in their avoidance of the agency, as both were caught within 'no man's land' between the definitions of a parent with care and a non-resident parent.

These two exemplary cases may not be typical of the CSA's client load. Where there is split residency of children and parents use the CSA's collection service, then the amount of maintenance to be paid is discretionary. But Rhidian was not clear how this might have operated in his case. The problem of proving paternity retrospectively is a policy issue and therefore beyond the brief of the CSA.

Rhidian's case highlights how his and the mother's behaviour in eluding the Agency may be construed as collusion. No such questions are raised by the behaviour of the remaining two fathers who avoided being assessed by the Agency. They cannot be accused of colluding with mothers – quite the reverse.

Coercion and avoidance

Both Lenny and Stephen had received a Maintenance Enquiry Form from the agency and this prompted them to seek further information on 'how much' their assessment was likely to be. Lenny's maintenance, previously arranged by the court, was to be increased substantially, while in Stephen's case it was to remain at a level similar to the amount he had agreed in private negotiations with the mother. Nonetheless both fathers responded similarly. They wanted to avoid CSA involvement and therefore both threatened to report the mothers for making fraudulent claims for Income Support. According to Lenny, the mother was working and not declaring her earnings and according to Stephen, the mother's partner was employed and his earnings were not being declared. Whether this was true or not, both mothers responded to these threats by withdrawing their claims for Income Support and the CSA subsequently dropped their cases. Lenny and Stephen continued to pay their maintenance at the previous levels. Lenny's concerns about the CSA were straightforward: he felt he could not afford the amount expected. Stephen, however, had other concerns.

Of the two, Stephen was initially more receptive to having his maintenance assessed by the CSA. But the turning point came when he realised that the amount he would have to pay was the exact same amount the mother was receiving in Income Support. He described his conversation with the CSA staff over this issue as follows:

> So what *you* are saying is *my* child support isn't just to cover for *my* child, it's to cover for his mum, his brother [the mothers' child to

her boyfriend], and her boyfriend, because he's out of work, so *I am* looking after the family.

Clearly Stephen's concerns were not related primarily to the amount he had to pay, but the distortion of his financial responsibilities brought about through the interaction between the CSA and the welfare benefits system. As the maintenance due was the same amount as Income Support, the system would in effect turn Stephen into the main breadwinner of the mother's new family and thereby alter his status as the financial provider for his son. Though the effect of his maintenance payments under a voluntary agreement may have been exactly the same (that each pound paid in maintenance would be deducted from Income Support) Stephen still placed a different meaning onto his CSA assessment. He said the CSA was unfair because:

> You know they are not just asking for child support, they are wanting to get as much money out of that person as they can so that the Government can pay as little as possible. I am totally against that.

Thus the problem identified by Stephen was the same as that identified by Peter above, that is the overlap between public and private responsibilities for non-resident children. But it was more complex than a simple juxtaposition of private responsibilities with the responsibility of the state to provide a subsistence income for children. The CSA assessment procedures effectively cut across the private responsibilities of stepfathers to maintain their own families and households. This raises more fundamental problems about child support policy itself, particularly the granting of a maintenance disregard for mothers dependent on Income Support.

It has been demonstrated how the lack of a maintenance disregard can be detrimental to children's welfare in the case of Peter. But additionally Peter and Stephen's cases highlight how the lack of a disregard distorts the private responsibilities of families. It is easy to imagine how this could work as a powerful disincentive for fathers (and perhaps mothers) to comply with the CSA. In this small sample of non-resident fathers there was no real evidence that parents were colluding to avoid their maintenance liability. It is possible that some policy makers might even be pleased about the behaviour of Lenny and Stephen, as they appeared to root out what they believed to be potential benefit fraud. However, such behaviour does raise concerns. If coercive tactics are applied by fathers in other circumstances, where mothers have no choice but to be dependent on Income Support for example, then the welfare of mothers and children may suffer. Whether the introduction of a maintenance disregard would be enough to alleviate these problems is open to question. Some people might argue that all the money paid in maintenance should go to children. This, however, would require a radical rethink of child support policy and welfare provision and would necessarily involve much philosophical debate about the roles of non-resident fathers, the roles of stepfathers and the role of the state. Such issues were not fully debated in the early proposals for a child support policy. Instead the Child Support Act 1991 romped home on the back of an over-simplistic belief that all fathers should pay maintenance. Most of the fathers in this second qualitative study agreed with the principle that they 'should pay' maintenance, but this espoused belief did not match everybody's behaviour and the reasons for this are explored in the next two chapters.

SUMMARY

The many changes that have been made to the child support system since the Child Support Act 1991 began to operate in April 1993 mean that some of the results of this research relating to the operation of the Child Support Agency may have only historical significance. Less than half of the non-resident fathers in the sample survey had had contact with the CSA at the time they were interviewed and only just over half of those had received a final or interim assessment. Of those who had received an assessment, not all had had to pay more maintenance as a result of it – in a quarter of the cases the amount that they were asked to pay actually went down. A third of those with a final assessment and three-quarters of those with an interim assessment had not started paying the amounts asked.

The majority of the fathers with a CSA assessment thought that it was unfair, most commonly because it did not take sufficient account of their living expenses. There was some evidence in the survey of the possible behavioural consequences of the CSA assessments. Of those assessed, 61 per cent thought that it would have an impact on their present living standard. Just over half the fathers expected that the assessment would affect for the worse their personal relations with their last partner, with their current partner or their non-resident children. Some of the fathers (18 per cent) feared that it might lead to a breakdown in the relationship with their new partner. A third said that it would lead to a reduction in informal payments of gifts for their children.

Substantial minorities thought it would have an impact on their labour supply or their willingness to repartner and become a father again.

These possible behavioural responses to the CSA assessments have been much neglected in discussions about the policy. Lowerson (1997) found that CSA assessments affect the labour supply behaviour of unemployed men by increasing their reservation wage and Clarke, Craig and Glendinning (1996a) found that the impact on relationships may be quite profound.

The qualitative study provided some further, though limited, insights into how behavioural changes could be produced. Most importantly, the child support system overlapped with the welfare benefit system in such away that it could distort the private financial responsibilities of fathers for their non-resident children. For example, in circumstances where the mothers had gone on to develop a second new family, and that family ended up dependent on Income Support, then the non-resident fathers felt they had replaced the stepfather as the breadwinner of that family. The maintenance they were expected to pay through the CSA could be equivalent to the sum received through Income Support. Thus one hitherto hidden consequence of the child support system is to interlink the financial responsibilities of stepfathers and non-resident fathers and thereby produce a strong reluctance to comply with the Agency. Note that this is not synonymous with a reluctance to pay maintenance, but specifically to pay maintenance under this system. Whether the behavioural consequences are collusive practices worked out with mothers is highly questionable. Indeed, if the responses of some of these men is typical, it is possible that some mothers and children are suffering financially as a result, especially if they feel forced to withdraw their claims for Income Support to appease the non-resident father and maintain cross-household family relationships.

The Child Support Act 1991 was based on the principle that biological fathers have an absolute and unreserved obligation to provide financial support for their children throughout their lives. Not all fathers accept this obligation and the reasons for this are discussed in Chapter 11.

11 Willingness to pay

INTRODUCTION

The quantitative study has provided information on the factors that affect maintenance payments, including information on the financial capacity of these respondents to meet their maintenance obligation. Obviously if fathers have limited financial means, they will be unable to pay maintenance, or much maintenance, but it has been argued that capacity to pay is closely related to willingness to pay (Burgoyne and Millar, 1994). For example, if maintenance payments can be given without incurring a high financial cost, this might increase willingness to pay; the converse also applies. However, what is not known is how other factors, less involved with financial capacity, are implicated in reaching a decision to pay. As Finch and Mason (1990) point out, there are no clear 'guidelines' to assist in the handling of post-divorce (and post-cohabiting and never lived together) relationships. This is particularly pertinent in cross-household financial transfers involving child maintenance payments. Yet competing views on the behaviour of non-resident fathers abound.

Fathers were portrayed by politicians as being 'irresponsible' and by policy makers as 'absent' parents. Contrary to this view, Families Need Fathers (FNF) (a fathers' rights group) portrayed fathers as innocent victims of circumstances with regard to their children.

> 'Absent Parents' *may* care very much and in no way have chosen to be 'absent' . . . 'their [fathers'] nurturing role must cover contact and residence (access and custody), as well as merely 'footing the bill'.
> (Families Need Fathers, 1990, para. 3)

Conceivably it suited policy makers to portray non-resident fathers in a negative way because this gave greater credence to a policy designed to make men pay – a point made by Finch (1989) in another context. On the other hand, it suited some men's purposes to oppose the legislation on economic grounds and/or on the grounds that they were purely victims of circumstances and therefore could not be held responsible. Importantly, FNF are a group of fathers who are working to ensure that fathers' contact with children following separation can be guaranteed more effectively by the legal system. They therefore represent one particular view. But what of other fathers in different circumstances – those with contact as well as those with no contact? One of the reasons for taking a qualitative approach was to give fathers, in different circumstances, 'a voice' to enable them to be heard above the loud chorus emanating from fathers in the anti-Act campaign groups. Some might well argue that fathers have already made their 'voices' heard. But contrary to this, it must be argued that their 'voice' has only had a selective hearing. As Smart (1989) asserts, the exercise of power within the law can act to disqualify different accounts of social reality. Indeed in the Social Security Committee's second inquiry into the operation of the 1991 Child Support Act, they ignored the viewpoint of fathers where they argued that their financial obligations should be conditional under certain circumstances (House of Commons, 470, 1994). The aim of giving fathers 'a voice' is therefore to facilitate an understanding of their social reality, as opposed to a perceived reality being promulgated by either politicians, the political process or single-issue pressure groups.

Correspondingly in trying to understand fathers' actions in regard to their parental obligations, there is also a need to contextualise their individual experiences. Qualitative in-depth interviews are best suited to achieve an understanding of how people's individual actions are both informed by, and are reflected back on their own frames of reference. Only by exploring people's attitudes, norms and behaviour – in other words their frames of reference – can an interpretation of people's actions be made (Allen and Skinner, 1991).

A qualitative approach is also appropriate where the uncovering of underlying processes and mechanisms is desired, and where the need for an 'insider' perspective is apparent (Bryman, 1992). The process of negotiation has been identified as a possible mechanism involved in fathers making commitments to children (discussed in the next chapter). This therefore requires further examination within a qualitative approach. Also, when considering the need for an insider perspective, one of the main dimensions that needs exploration is fathers' 'willingness to pay' maintenance, and how this willingness relates to fathers' perceptions of the 'affordability' of maintenance. This can only be understood from the 'inside', from the respondents' perspective and will thus complement the quantitative survey's assessment of capacity to pay, providing a fuller understanding of willingness to pay.

The overall purpose of this qualitative study is therefore to delve deeper into the financial obligations of non-residential fathers to cast some light on how commitments to pay maintenance are developed, sustained and sometimes dissolved, and will thus seek to discover why some men pay maintenance while others do not. The more specific questions addressed in this chapter are, first, how do fathers both view and enact their social and moral obligation to their non-resident children within the context of their own lives? Second, what factors militate against or facilitate fathers' willingness to pay maintenance and how are these related to one another? We begin by describing the characteristics of the eighteen respondents in this qualitative subsample.

RESPONDENT CHARACTERISTICS

Eighteen non-resident fathers were interviewed in depth. The fathers' ages ranged between 29 and 52 years. Ten of the eighteen were employed, three of whom were self-employed, with two owning their own businesses (Table 11.1). Occupations among the employed included: two lorry drivers, bereavement counsellor, social worker, prison officer, bar manager, taxi driver and insurance broker. The two businesses were a contract cleaning firm and a plumbing firm. Of the remaining eight, five were unemployed and dependent upon social security benefits, two were students and one had taken early retirement.

Table 11.1 Employment status

Employed	7
Self-employed	3
Unemployed	5
Retired	1
Student	2
Total respondents	18

Non-resident children

All the fathers had at least one dependent non-resident child for whom there was a legal obligation to pay maintenance (Table 11.2). A dependent child is defined as under the age of 16 or between 16 and 18 and in full-time education. However, five fathers had two sets of non-resident children from two past relationships. In three of those cases the children from first past families were now adult and the obligation to provide child maintenance had therefore ceased. This leaves twenty past relationships involving dependent children and in the subsequent analysis these relationships are examined independently. Thus, there are twenty past relationships but only eighteen fathers. These multiple relationships are referred to as the first past relationship (1) and the second (2) past relationship; the second relationship was the most recent.

Table 11.2 Number of past relationships and number of non-resident children

No. of past relationships	
One past relationship	13
Two past relationships	5
Total past relationships	23
No. of non-resident children	
Fathers with one child	11
Fathers with two children	5★
Fathers with three children	2
Total non-resident children	27

★ Contains two cases where fathers had one child in each of two past relationships.

Second families

Some of these eighteen respondents had developed new family relationships: seven were married currently and five were cohabiting (Table 11.3). Of those twelve repartnered fathers, six had new children to their current partner and three had stepchildren. Nine fathers therefore had responsibilities for children living in their households as well as having an obligation to pay child maintenance for their non-resident children. A more detailed description of each of the fathers' current relationships is provided within the findings.

Table 11.3 Second families

Married to new partner	7
Cohabiting	5
Single	6
Has new child in household	6
Has stepchildren in household	3
Child from past relationship	1

Table 11.4 Maintenance provision

Name	Maintenance arrangement	Paying now
Willing payment		
Alan	Voluntary agreement★	Yes
Theo	Court agreement	Yes
Lenny	Court agreement	Yes
Carlton	Court agreement	Yes
Matthew	Court agreement	Yes
Stephen	Voluntary agreement	Yes
Peter	CSA agreement★	Yes
Malcolm (2)	CSA and voluntary sum	Yes
Harold (2)	Voluntary agreement	Yes
Enforced payments		
Collin	Court attachment of earnings order	Yes
Robert	Court agreement	Yes
Paul	CSA agreement	Yes
Harold (1)	Court attachment of earnings	Yes
Non-payments		
Leo	Never had agreement	No – paid in past
Barry	CSA case in hand	Never paid
Malcolm (1)	No agreement★	No – paid in past
Ian	No agreement★	No – paid in past
Henry	CSA case in hand★★	No – paid in past
Rhidian	No agreement★	No – paid in past
Alex	Never had agreement	Never paid

★   Previously had court agreement.
★★ Previously paid lump sum in lieu of maintenance.
(1) first past relationship.
(2) second past relationship.

Payment of maintenance

In order to examine how financial commitments to pay maintenance were developed, the respondents were grouped according to whether they were paying maintenance or not. The payers were then subdivided into two groups, those who were paying as a result of enforcement and those who were apparently paying willingly. Although this is a crude categorisation, it allows comparisons to be made to ascertain how and under what circumstances maintenance payments were sustained or dissolved. Table 11.4 describes the types of maintenance agreements the fathers had, whether they were currently paying maintenance and whether these payments were enforced. The respondents are given pseudonyms with their agreement.

In all of the twenty past relationships thirteen fathers were currently paying maintenance and in four of these cases there was an element of enforcement attached to payment. The definition of enforcement was where fathers said that they would not have paid if the maintenance had not been deducted at source (attachment of earnings or directly from benefit entitlement) or there was not the threat of legal action for non-payment. In the seven other relationships no maintenance was currently being paid, but in five cases the fathers claimed to have paid in the past, one of whom said he gave a single cash payment at the time of separation (£60,000). Of the two fathers with multiple past relationships, both were currently paying maintenance for their children from second past partnerships, but only one of them (Harold) was paying maintenance for his child from his first relationship, which was enforced. In only four of the twenty relationships had there *never* been a formal agreement made through the courts, with solicitors or through the Child Support Agency. Yet maintenance payments were not dependent upon a formal agreement, and neither did the existence of a formal agreement guarantee payments. Stephen, and Harold in his second relationship, had always paid on a voluntary basis, and of the non-payers three had court agreements.

Analysis

This small group of men exhibit a wide variation in terms of their employment and occupational status, current family circumstances and maintenance payment status. Payment of itself, however, does not necessarily signify commitment, as four fathers had to have maintenance payments enforced. Similarly non-payment may not signify a lack of commitment, as Henry claimed to have paid a 'one off' lump sum in lieu of regular payments. Therefore to find out how these fathers did make commitments, the nine willing payers will be contrasted with the other two groups together, enforced and non-payers.

It is important to note that although the unit of analysis is the fathers themselves, they are actually grouped according to each of their past relationships. Thus Harold and Malcolm are willing payers regarding second past relationships but not in their first past relationships. Harold's payments were enforced for his child from his first past relationship and Malcolm paid nothing for his first child.

Additionally actual amounts of maintenance offered by individual fathers are not described systematically. The intention is to avoid creating a moral hierarchy in which fathers who are seen to be paying the highest amounts are equated with being the most committed to their children. As Finch argues, people feel able to make 'strong moral judgements' about other people's duties and obligations (Finch, 1989: 189).

This is something our analysis is keen to avoid, not only because amounts of maintenance will vary according to individual circumstances, but also because maintenance payments are but one form of support fathers can provide for their children. What is of interest to us is to explore how fathers become committed to paying maintenance and what sustains this commitment, rather than seek to make judgements about whether the amounts paid were adequate. We recognise that this is an important issue for mothers, children and policy makers. Nonetheless, the question addressed here asks what is it about the willing payers, or their circumstances, that influenced their payment of maintenance? How did these fathers perceive their financial capacity to pay maintenance and how important was this in influencing payment? In addressing these questions the current socio-economic circumstances of the willing payers are described first.

WILLING PAYERS

Socio-economic circumstances

Table 11.5 presents a summary of willing payers' current employment status and a history of their current and past family relationships. Only

Table 11.5 Current socio-economic circumstances of willing payers and the history of their past relationships

Name	Work status	No. of children in current family	Current marital status and time lived with current partner	Ages of non-resident children	Past marital status and time lived with mother	Contact with children
Alan	Retired	1	M 14yrs	23, 21, 17	M 13yrs	Yes
Theo	Self-employed	2*	M 4yrs	16	M 8yrs	Yes
Lenny	Employed	none	M 4yrs	15	M 10yrs	Yes
Carlton	Student	none	Single	17, 16	M 11yrs	Yes
Matthew	Employed	3*	M 18mths	14	M 18mths	No
Stephen	Employed	1 and[a]	M 5yrs	12	Cohabit 18mths	Yes
Peter	Employed	none	M 7yrs	16, 14, 12	M 9yrs	Yes
Malcolm (2)	Inactive	1* and[a]	Cohabit 2yrs	9	Cohabit 5yrs	Yes
Harold (2)	Employed	none	Single	5	Cohabit 5yrs	Yes

M = married.
* Stepchildren.
a Partner pregnant.

three of the nine were economically inactive. One was a student, the other retired and the other unemployed. Broadly this suggests that as a group there was some capacity to pay maintenance, but many had demands on their incomes from current families. Just how did these fathers perceive their maintenance obligation in this context?

Maintenance as a duty

The willing payers described maintenance payments as a 'duty', something that was 'owed', as part of the responsibility of bringing the child into the world, or as part of their responsibilities to their children. In that sense they 'owned' the responsibility, they accepted that the obligation to pay maintenance belonged to them.

Generally this acceptance of the obligation appeared to be unconditional. Typical comments included:

> I have got a financial responsibility to [child] and there is no question about that at all . . .

> it was sort of I have got to pay that and that's it, that is my duty . . .

> I thought an ongoing commitment in terms of maintenance was right . . .

For six of the willing payers this sense of duty seemed steadfast regardless of obligations to children in second families. They said their non-resident children 'came first' or 'equal first' with children in their current families. Therefore these six made no distinction between responsibilities for children within or outside their households, including stepchildren. The remaining three fathers, however, did *not* explicitly prioritise non-resident children.

Mathew said his stepchildren came first, Lenny said himself and his wife came first and Carlton felt his own needs took priority. Compared with the other six willing payers, these three were less involved with their non-resident children. Mathew, the only father in the willing group with no contact, had not seen his child for seven years. Lenny saw his child for only a couple of hours a fortnight, but he said this arrangement suited him. Carlton had infrequent contact over the years and felt that the children viewed him as 'unimportant' in their lives.

The different ordering of priorities therefore partly reflected the degree of involvement fathers had with their non-resident children.

Nonetheless despite this, and despite the presence of second families, all the willing payers accepted the obligation to pay maintenance and were doing so. This did not mean, however, that all found payments affordable.

Trying hard to pay maintenance

All the fathers described how they had struggled to maintain payments during periods of financial hardship. Such hardship was experienced in two main ways. First, the early period following separation was seen as particularly difficult. Second, unemployment or early retirement (in one case) was another difficult time. The period of resettlement following separation placed many financial burdens upon these respondents. For some this was due to foregoing their share of equity in the marital home, which meant they had to finance the purchase of another house from existing income only. Other factors like debts from the marriage or from failed businesses, and the legal costs of divorce were viewed as heavy financial burdens. However, as the period of resettlement ended and as the amounts of maintenance stayed relatively fixed over time, payments generally became more affordable. That is, if the father's stayed in employment. However, unemployment itself did not necessarily result in non-payment.

Three fathers who experienced unemployment said they *tried hard* to maintain payments during these times. For example, Carlton, who was currently a student, said he insisted on making a small weekly payment to the court, although the court did not expect payment due to his lack of earned income. Similarly, Lenny had kept payments going during repeated short episodes of unemployment. Malcolm said that although he was unemployed he 'earned money on the side' and it was this money he used to top up his CSA maintenance for his second child (see Table 11.4). This continued commitment to pay in the face of financial difficulty carried with it a sense of pride. Alan described this well:

> we managed to get through and for my own sort of self respect I was thinking whatever it was [the maintenance] I would pay that, try . . .

Yet despite improvement in some of these fathers' financial circumstances, the amounts paid were generally not increased over time. In only two cases had amounts been increased since the point of separation. It could be that maintenance was therefore generally affordable and this may have contributed to willingness to pay. Equally, however, when the fathers were unemployed, they kept payments going. Fluctuations in income therefore seemed to have little impact on whether maintenance was paid or not (at least over the short-term – six months or so). This suggests both a strong commitment to pay among the willing payers and that financial capacity to pay was not the main factor in developing and sustaining this commitment. However, this apparently unconditional commitment to pay must be understood within the context of relationships with mothers and children and the *usefulness* of maintenance in these relationships.

RELATIONSHIPS WITH MOTHERS AND CHILDREN

Useful maintenance

With the exception of Matthew, the rest of the willing payers had active contact with their children, though not all had friendly relationships with mothers. Nonetheless, contact helped sustain their commitment because maintenance payments were useful in these relationships. For example, Theo said he paid because:

> it just made it oil the wheels easier that's all to make sure there was no ups and downs of access or anything like that . . .

For Theo, his maintenance worked as a kind of guarantee for contact. But he also stated that he paid it to make sure 'they' [the mother and son] would not be 'hard up financially' and that it was to make up for 'not being there' as a father living in his son's household. Theo's commitment was therefore underpinned by a multiplicity of reasons: to ensure his son's well-being, as a lever for ensuring contact and to compensate his son for the absence of his father in his daily life. Similarly, the other willing payers explicitly gave multiple reasons for paying maintenance, which included: paying maintenance in recognition of the mothers' daily caring responsibilities, to persuade or even coerce the mother into agreeing to contact and to ensure the children's financial well-being. One father even likened maintenance payments to a wage for the mother as the resident parent.

Paying maintenance could therefore help keep the relationship with the mother in balance. It could represent the father's parental contribution to offset the mother's daily caring responsibilities – almost a clear division of labour; or payments could operate on a reciprocal basis where fathers expected contact with children in return for payment. However, payments could also be given in recognition of the child's entitlement, or given as compensation to make up for some perceived lack by the father. The particular mix of reasons given for payment varied on an individual basis, but these were the common themes. These proffered reasons expose how relationships with mothers and with children overlapped within the maintenance obligation. The mothers could receive maintenance based on their own entitlement as the primary carer. Additionally they show how in these particular relationships some fathers could gain from payment – receiving contact with their children. However, guilt was also a factor in motivating willing payers, though they did not give this as an explicit reason themselves. Matthew, who had no contact with his child, did gain some relief from his sense of guilt through paying maintenance – even though he did not gain contact.

Matthew

Matthew was consumed with guilt about his decision to end his relationship with the mother when his son was only six months old. Additionally, he felt he had behaved irresponsibly over contact arrangements. When his son was a baby, Matthew said he did not want the responsibility of looking after him at weekends. However, as his son grew older Matthew became more reliable over contact visits until he lost contact altogether subsequent to two interrelated events. The mother moved 200 miles away and Matthew's relationship with her and with her boyfriend deteriorated. Consequently, Matthew had not seen his son for the last seven years. In this context he described his current responsibility to his son as follows:

> That I should love him purely as a father should.

and he went on to define this as:

> I see that I still owe [ex-wife] or [son] if you like eh a duty to em see that he doesn't go without to certain respects. . . . My responsibility to him now is purely a financial one.

Paying maintenance was, as Matthew said, an expression of his fatherly love. Paying was therefore meaningful for Matthew, as it helped bolster his self-identity as a responsible and caring father. However, he also felt his maintenance was a duty *owed* to the mother, as he was ashamed that he had left her to cope alone when his son was just a baby. It was therefore Matthew's sense of shame and guilt that underpinned his commitment to pay. Having a sense of guilt about past events was evident among four of the other willing payers.

Alleviating guilt

Three fathers (Alan, Peter and Lenny) had committed adultery and left the family home to live with their mistresses, whom they all eventually married. They did not regret divorcing their wives, but they did regret the disruption this caused to their children's family life. All three expressed feelings of guilt about the emotional and psychological harm caused to children as a consequence of them departing from the family home. The fathers said they 'dreaded' the day when their children might hold them to account for their actions. However, feelings of guilt did not stem only from fathers' adulterous behaviour. One other father, Carlton, felt guilty that he had not tried hard enough to save his marriage (his wife had the affair). Carlton perceived that his relationship with his children had deteriorated enormously subsequent to the difficulties he experienced in parenting them as a non-resident father. Though these four men expressed feelings of guilt about past events and their consequences, they did not overtly give this as a reason for paying maintenance. Rather, as already highlighted, they described their maintenance obligation in terms of a 'duty owed', or in terms of it being 'right' that they should pay. It is possible that this sense of duty was born out of feelings of guilt, as feeling guilty implies a desire to take some responsibility for one's actions. Thus, despite their description of maintenance as an unconditional duty, this may not have been the case. They may have felt it their duty to pay maintenance because they wanted to *compensate* children and possibly mothers for their past behaviour within these family relationships. This could explain why they persevered with payments even when they found it financially difficult and why they had either *prioritised* their maintenance obligation and/or had *selected* themselves as the ones who should fulfil this responsibility. Guilt could therefore act as a precondition for payment.

The behaviour and attitudes of the willing payers fit within a normative expectation that parents should be altruistic towards their children and that fathers 'should pay' some maintenance even if this involves an element of self-sacrifice. Does this mean, therefore, that the enforced payers and non-payers are inherently irresponsible or selfish individuals? Possibly not, as Harold and Malcolm were paying maintenance willingly in their second past relationships (examined here), but not in their first past relationships. So what was it about the enforced payment and non-payment relationships that could help explain reluctance to pay or non-payment? To address this question the socio-economic circumstances of these two groups and the history of their past relationships are described first.

ENFORCED PAYERS AND NON-PAYERS

Socio–economic circumstances

Table 11.6 demonstrates that more of the enforced payers and non-payers were economically inactive (six), compared with the willing payers (two). Though obviously Malcolm and Harold's current circumstances remain the same for their first and second past relationships, the former are examined here. Four fathers also had second families to support (as

Table 11.6 Socio-economic circumstances of enforced payers and non-payers and the history of past relationships

Name	Work status	No. of children in current family	Current marital status and time lived with current partner	Ages of non-resident children	Past marital status and time lived with mother	Contact with children
Enforced payers						
Collin	Employed	1	Cohabit 4yrs	8	M 18mths	No
Robert	Employed	2	M 5yrs	17	M 10yrs	No
Paul	Inactive	None	Single	7	M 8yrs	No
Harold (1)	Employed	None	Single	9	Never lived with mother	No
Non-payers						
Leo	Inactive	None	Single	14	Never lived with mother	No
Barry	Employed	None	Cohabit 3mths	7, 5	M 5yrs	Yes
Malcolm (1)	Inactive	1★ª	Cohabit 2yrs	11	M 2yrs	No
Ian	Inactive	None	Single	8	M 6yrs	No
Henry	Employed	1	Cohabit 6yrs	12, 9	M 10yrs	No
Rhidian	Student	1ᵇ	Lone parent	13ᵇ	M 6yrs	No
Alex	Inactive	1	Cohabit 18mths	6★★	Cohabit 3yrs	No

M = married
a   Partner pregnant
b   This father had split residency of his children; his son lived with him and the daughter with the mother.
★   Stepchild
★★ The mother denied this respondent was the father of this child.

did four within the willing group). One other father, Rhidian, was simultaneously a non-resident parent and a lone parent, as he had residency of his son and the mother had residency of their daughter. The most striking feature of all these relationships was the lack of contact fathers had with their non-resident children. Only one of the eleven fathers had contact. This was the exact opposite of the willing payers, where only one father did *not* have contact. Before exploring the issue of contact further, the question of how capacity to pay maintenance may have influenced these fathers' perceptions of their maintenance obligation needs addressing.

Capacity to pay

In none of the enforced payment or non-paying relationships did the fathers prioritise their financial obligations to non-resident children. Where fathers had second families, these resident children were deemed to 'come first', and the fathers without resident children said their own needs came first. This lack of financial priority given to non-resident children was partly explained by the poor economic circumstances of some of these fathers. However, this was not as straightforward as it might appear, as changing life events were interlinked in a complex way with poor economic circumstances.

Changing life events

Three of the six unemployed fathers had stopped paying maintenance as a result of certain dramatic incidents. The sudden change of residency of one of Rhidian's two children prompted a new agreement with the mother to halt maintenance payments. Ian had attempted suicide; this action had many immediate consequences. He lost his job and he lost contact with his daughter; consequently he also stopped paying maintenance. Leo was accused of sexually abusing his child and immediately lost contact. He no longer knew where his child lived and as he had paid maintenance direct to the mother during visits, he therefore ceased to pay once contact was lost. Thus, though there was a limited capacity to pay maintenance, this was also not the *right time* in these men's lives to pay.

Among the remaining eight relationships, other factors that contributed to it not being the right time to pay maintenance included: the previous payment of a lump sum for maintenance, the repaying of debts incurred within the marriage or resulting from divorce, the existence of second families and paying maintenance for other children (Malcolm and Harold). It was difficult to prioritise the maintenance obligation to these particular children in such circumstances. However, it was not just the fathers' own socio-economic circumstances that contributed to the low priority given to the maintenance obligation, but the mothers' as well.

Selecting others

Among the enforced payment and non-paying relationships the fathers tended to select others to carry the financial responsibilities of parenthood. They felt it was the mother's and her partner's responsibility to meet the financial needs of children (seven of the eleven mothers were known to have repartnered). For some fathers this was born out of a belief (true or false) that the mother's household income was greater than their own. For example, Ian said:

> I mean to be honest I felt once she had remarried and they were both working and I was out of work I thought hang on a minute, why should I have that uh responsibility for [daughter's] you know basic needs when she [mother] has chosen to take – she remarried, they have got two loads of savings – why am I still having to pay so much?

In fact Ian had never paid maintenance when he was unemployed. What he was referring to was a period of particular financial difficulties when he sought a reduction in his maintenance through the courts (unsuccessfully). Nevertheless his statement highlights his sense of unfairness at paying maintenance when the mother was believed to be better off than himself. Thus, the mother and/or the stepfather were selected to shoulder the financial responsibilities of parenthood on the basis of this guideline of *financial equity* across the two households. Five other fathers used this guideline of financial equity to rationalise their reluctance to pay maintenance.

Thus we see how these fathers gave a low priority to the maintenance obligation. They either needed the money for themselves/second families, or they felt their non-resident children did not need maintenance, or they believed that at this moment in time, the financial responsibility now lay with the mother and her partner, if she had one. On these grounds the fathers found the obligation to pay unacceptable. First, economically there was a restricted capacity to pay because of low incomes, unemployment or overlapping and competing demands from current families. Second, there were the factors of time and change; mental illness, changes of residency of children, loss of contact, and economic debts resulting from family dissolution – all affected how these fathers prioritised the maintenance obligation.

Yet if the enforced payers and non-payers are compared with the willing payers, then this lack of commitment to pay maintenance is not fully explained by poor economic circumstances alone. Fathers in the willing paying group still managed to pay maintenance even where they had second families and when they were financially hard pressed. Some even paid while recognising that the mother's household income was greater than their own. So just why was the obligation to pay less acceptable within the enforced payment and non-paying relationships? The answer lies partly in the history of the relationship with mothers and the fathers' sense of loss and marginalisation in their children's lives. As already highlighted, all, except Barry, had no contact with their children. How did this affect commitment to pay maintenance?

RELATIONSHIPS WITH MOTHERS AND CHILDREN

Hostility and loss

A powerful feature of these enforced payment and non-paying relationships was the hostility fathers felt towards mothers. Some of this hostility presented itself as resentment about past financial matters. Mothers were described at the very least as materialistic and selfish, if not actually callous thieves, hell-bent on 'bleeding' fathers 'dry'. Such criticisms of mothers were not entirely absent within the willing paying relationships, but for the enforced payers and non-payers these criticisms exemplified the fathers' continued resentments about the history of relationships with mothers. Depending on the individual case, this could include the following:

- feelings of loss over the failure of the adults' relationship (six cases);
- loss of the fathers' relationships with children (all excluding Harold);
- loss of the family home and everything that the father had worked for (four cases);
- anger at the mother's apparent adultery (five cases);
- anger at being left with debts following relationship breakdown (five cases);
- anger at perceived financial inequity between mothers' and fathers' households (five cases);
- loss of the biological status of father through denial of paternity by the mother (Alex only); and
- anger at having no say in becoming a father in the first instance (Harold only).

Regarding these particular past relationships, all the enforced payers and non-payers were hurt, confused, frustrated and/or angry. Even where the particular events giving rise to these feelings had happened years previously, this had generally not been ameliorated with the passage of time. Indeed the experience of recalling events for interview purposes created considerable distress for some. This is perhaps indicative of what Kruk (1992) found among his respondents: that where fathers had lost contact with their children, they were still in the grieving process. Certainly the majority wanted contact with their children but had been unable to achieve this. However, one father, Harold, had never wanted contact with his child.

Harold's relationship with the mother of his first child had been very fleeting: he had been unaware that she was pregnant and was not involved in any decision to continue the pregnancy. His animosity towards this mother was almost palpable. This was partly because maintenance payments had been enforced by the courts. Harold said he did not care if the amount paid 'was too much or too little', all he wanted to do was 'buy off' the mother – 'to get her out of his life forever'. To that end he offered her a sum of £10,000. In return she was to sign an affidavit to release him from the maintenance obligation, but she refused. Such bargaining with mothers over the maintenance obligation was exceptional. Harold was the only respondent who dismissed outright any financial obligation to pay maintenance. However, such dismissal was restricted to this child from his first past relationship; as already discussed, he paid maintenance willingly for his second child. Nonetheless, it shows how hostility towards mothers spilled over into financial obligations. For the rest in the enforced payment and non-payment groups it tended to manifest itself in mistrust over how mothers might spend maintenance monies.

Squandered maintenance

The issue of how the mothers might spend maintenance monies was a deeply felt concern for six of the seven non-payers and one of the four enforced payers. They believed maintenance payments would be squandered as the money would be spent on improving the mother's and/or her boyfriend's life-style. A particular focus of concern for four of them was the potential use of maintenance monies on a car. It did not matter whether it was used for the purchase of a car or to meet its running costs; it still rankled. Maintenance spent on a car was not seen to be of value to children, only of value to the mother and, worse still, of value to her new husband/boyfriend.

Other variations on this theme were where fathers felt maintenance would be spent on cigarettes, alcohol, nights out for the mother and decorating the house and so on. All these items were specifically picked to prove how the mothers' control over spending could not guarantee that children would benefit from maintenance payments. In that sense fathers would not get *value for money*.

However, only Henry (the non-payer who claimed to have given a cash lump sum in lieu of regular maintenance) seemed to have evidence that the maintenance had been *squandered*. He accused the mother of 'blowing the money' on holidays abroad and on boyfriends. He was annoyed that the lump sum of £60,000, given six years previously, had all gone and the mother and children were now dependent on Income Support. The others, however, had little evidence that maintenance payments had been or would be squandered. Yet they knew for a 'fact' that maintenance would not be spent on children. To prove this 'fact' many examples of the mothers' selfishness were cited. These examples served as *atrocity stories* about mothers (Silverman, 1993). The construction of atrocity stories was used to highlight how the mothers were pernicious, calculating and money-grabbing. It was pointless to pay maintenance to a person who would only use the money for their own ends. Thus, a double jeopardy was attached to maintenance payments. The mothers could spend it inappropriately (on cars, holidays and so on), but in addition their innate selfishness would ensure that their own needs would come first before the children's.

Demonising mothers

The seven fathers also told atrocity stories about mothers to demonstrate how she was the one who took the children, who would go to any lengths to stop contact, and who rejected or ejected the father. According to the fathers, the 'lengths' that the mothers 'would go to' included:

- 'false' accusations of child sex abuse;
- telling the child their father was dead;
- 'brain washing' the children against their fathers;
- 'disappearing' without warning and not sending a forwarding address;

and less dramatically:

- refusing to meet fathers 'half way' metaphorically or physically in enabling contact with children.

Thus, it was the mothers' behaviour towards them as fathers that was atrocious in the eyes of these men. Typically the fathers commented that they 'could not put into words' how they felt about the mothers. These atrocity stories served to display several things: a deep sense of loss, of powerlessness and victimisation in their role as fathers, and the unfairness and pointlessness of paying maintenance when they were being denied satisfactory relationships with their children. For in the post-separation period, none of these men would accept responsibility for failed relationships. Though they grudgingly admitted that their own behaviour may have contributed to failed relations, they remained bemused about how this had led to such dire consequences of loss of contact with children. Transgressions such as not turning up for pre-arranged contact visits, or failing to communicate between visits that may have been three months apart, were not deemed big enough to produce such critical outcomes. Even the attempted suicide of one father was viewed by him as irrelevant. Evidence from Kruk (1992) in part supports these findings; he claims that on the whole fathers tended to underestimate their own role in regards to loss of contact (p. 86). From Kruk's viewpoint the role played by fathers in lost contact was due to the negative consequences of an abnormal grieving process brought about by the loss of children and the loss of the pre-divorce father–child relationship. It is difficult to say how far this grieving process affected these fathers in our study, though this may have been a significant factor in Ian's attempted suicide. For the others it is more likely that they were unable or unwilling to assess how their 'unreliability' over contact arrangements could be detrimental to developing a new contract of trust with the mother and/or children. As Goto (1996) points out, the relationship aspect of trust involves relying on the character, strength, or truth of someone and is synonymous with co-operation (p. 120). Clearly the atrocity stories demonstrated a deep suspicion and a complete lack of faith in mothers as co-parents.

Nonetheless, demonising mothers was the only way these fathers could make sense of their lack of involvement in their children's lives. Furthermore if fathers were to focus on the part they had played in failed relationships, they would have undermined the credibility of their atrocity stories. Simpson *et al.* (1995) found similar responses among the non-resident fathers in their sample who had no contact with their children. In their study they commented on the fathers' use of words:

> 'assassination', 'crucifixion', and 'poisoning' used by some fathers bring to mind a slow and lingering death: in this instance the death

is that of fatherhood and it is the custodial mother who is felt to wield power over life and death.

(p. 33)

However, among the enforced payers and non-payers in this study, in discussion about child maintenance, the whole point of these atrocity stories was to prove innocence and therefore justify reluctance or non-payment of maintenance.

Contact and maintenance

In reality these fathers in the non-paying and enforced payment groups saw their maintenance obligation as primarily a payment made to the mother. They questioned why they should pay maintenance to the mother when she would not reciprocate by 'allowing' them some parental responsibilities in terms of caring. Clearly there was an expectation for mothers to ease the fathers' relationships with their children. What the atrocity stories signify is that not only were the mothers apparently failing to meet this expectation, but that the fathers could not understand why this was so. The 'proper thing for the mother to do' was to enable contact, while the 'proper thing for the father to do' was to pay maintenance. This exposes the 'silent bargain' attached to maintenance payments. The clearest example of this came from one enforced payer, Robert. His story highlights what can happen when reciprocal relations break down.

Robert explicitly objected to paying maintenance when he had no contact:

> The things I begrudged was the fact that I was paying it after a while and having no contact. The very fact of paying maintenance that didn't bother me. If I'd had contact I would have paid double that, but you just get resentful after a while, with no contact when you are still paying; paying for a child you aren't seeing.

Robert responded to his resentment by repeatedly withholding maintenance till the court stepped in to enforce it. He described this behaviour as 'childish'. But he said that it was his way of making a 'protest' to the mother; he wanted her to respond by agreeing to contact. However, his protest was also a means through which he could relay his anger, frustration and sense of loss about his relationship with his son:

Just having no contact you don't realise what it is, what it involves. You go through a period of bereavement I suppose . . . it's just like having – or similar to having – a death of a child, that's the only way I could describe it.

He went on to say:

You could break down and cry, I have many times, then you get all resentful towards it if you like and hardened to it. . . . You realise that you are not going to get it [contact] and you get . . . you can't get it away from your mind.

So powerful were Robert's feelings that his disruptive behaviour and protest lasted for six years. He finally complied with payments on time when he had only two years left to pay.

SUMMARY

The key difference between the groups was the lack of, or presence of, contact with non-resident children. All of the willing payers, bar one, had contact and they had selected themselves as having a *duty* or *obligation* to pay maintenance (even if they did not always place their obligations to non-resident children first). The act of paying maintenance was also useful and/or meaningful to them in their relationships with children and for their personal identity as fathers. Payment could work as a guarantee for contact with children by '*easing*' relationships with mothers or as a tool to manipulate mothers into agreeing to contact arrangements. Payment could also act to compensate children and/or mothers for a past misdemeanour, or for some perceived lack by the father. All these factors helped the willing payers develop and sustain commitments to paying maintenance. Such commitments were held so strongly that some fathers were determined to pay even when unemployed.

We have suggested that feeling guilty was a possible pre-condition for developing a commitment to pay within some of the willing payers' relationships. This was evident in the ways that fathers paid maintenance on a compensatory basis. Victimisation, on the other hand, was the converse of guilt. A sense of victimisation or blamelessness was the overriding feeling exhibited by most of the enforced payers and non-payers. The majority had no contact with their children and felt that the mothers were at least unsupportive, if not obstructive, in facilitating the father–child relationship. In these relationships the enforced payers and non-payers could not, or would not, acknowledge any responsibility for failed relationships post-separation, that is apart from Harold, who did not want contact with his first child. The rest were confused and angry about their lack of satisfactory relationships with children. Such negative feelings did not form a sound basis from which to begin to accept the maintenance obligation. The enforced payers and non-payers tended *not* to accept that there was a legitimate 'need' for this kind of financial support. Either their own or second families' financial needs were a *priority*, or the mothers (and stepfathers) were *selected* as having the financial capacity or obligation to meet the costs of parenting unsupported by the father. Moreover, they believed that even if they did pay, this money would simply be squandered by mothers. Making payments therefore served no useful purpose, as it could not be used to facilitate contact with children, despite sustained attempts by some (as exemplified by Robert) to use it in this way. Nor did it alleviate guilt where fathers felt victimised. Ultimately they rejected the obligation primarily upon failed *reciprocal* relations with mothers; if mothers would not 'allow' contact, then why should the fathers pay maintenance? Given the importance of relationships with mothers and children in the development and sustenance of financial commitments, this suggests that the maintenance obligation was negotiated. This process of negotiation is discussed in the next chapter.

12 Negotiating child maintenance

INTRODUCTION

In Chapter 11 we explored the factors that impinged upon fathers' 'willingness to pay' and how this helped sustain financial commitments. But this does not tell us about the processes and mechanisms that underlie the development or otherwise of these commitments. To explore these we need to engage with theoretical debates on family obligations and financial obligations. The theoretical underpinnings to the study are therefore viewed as being twofold: first, the processes involved in making financial commitments to help support family members and, second, the relationship between obligations and money. On obligations and money Finch (1989) has argued that policy that defines people's financial obligations may fail if that policy is out of line with what people regard as fair. An earlier example of this was the demise of the Poll Tax. Finch and Mason (1993) in their work on family obligations have identified that adults work out what support they will give through a process of negotiation rather than through fixed rules such as those implied by duty or obligation. Similarly, people do not expect that others have a right to make claims upon them for support. Commitments are therefore created within a process of negotiation where people accept or reject their responsibility to give support in the light of their specific circumstances. Responsibilities are therefore the products of negotiated commitments developed over time (Finch and Mason, 1993: 179).

Finch and Mason's work was, however, restricted to exploring commitments between adult kin and therefore the framework of negotiated commitments might seem an inappropriate way of exploring non-resident fathers' obligations to their *dependent* children. The moral duty on fathers (and all parents) to provide financially for dependent children is so strong that it is surely non-negotiable, a principle upheld by the Child Support Acts. Children as dependants have a right to expect this support, not least because their needs are immediate. They cannot wait for their fathers (or mothers) to develop commitments to them over time. However, non-resident fathers enact their obligations against a background of family fragmentation. They therefore have at least two sets of social relations and obligations to consider: those with children *and* with mothers (more if they have second families). These two primary sets of relations have been described as representing a simultaneous continuity and discontinuity. Fathers may want a continuing relationship with children, but within the context of a discontinued relationship with the mother (Simpson *et al.*, 1995). There is therefore a schism in these two primary sets of relationships and the interesting question is whether and how this schism creates a negotiated commitment. But making financial commitments also involves giving money and it is unknown how the medium of money might impact further on developing commitments to pay child maintenance. In this chapter we will explore both of these factors. We begin by reviewing the evidence already presented in Chapter 11 to see how commitments to pay may have been developed within a process of negotiation. To do that we need to understand, first, how negotiations operate in practice.

OPERATING NEGOTIATIONS

In describing how the process of negotiation operates, Finch and Mason (1990) argue that people apply certain moral guidelines to steer them in negotiations. Thus, people apply moral principles such as fairness and justice in negotiations; this helps guide their conduct in negotiations. But in addition they apply more specific normative guidelines to work out what to do in practice. The normative guidelines identified by Finch (1989) are where: people prioritise across all their responsibilities; they select whether they are the appropriate person to give the support based on the past history of the relationship with that person; they assess the past patterns of reciprocal exchange with that person, striving to maintain a balance between independence and dependence; and they assess whether it is the right time in their lives to give support of the kind asked (p. 178).

If these normative guidelines are applied to the findings already presented in Chapter 11, then there is evidence that the financial obligations were negotiated. Fathers did prioritise their financial obligations, select others to financially support their non-resident children, decide it was not the right time in their lives to pay maintenance and based their willingness to pay, at least in part, on reciprocal exchanges with mothers, particularly over contact with children. For example, the willing payers, most of whom had contact, found their maintenance payments useful in maintaining contact with children as it 'eased' relationships with mothers. These payments therefore helped balance reciprocal exchanges with mothers and fathers were willing to pay.

Conversely, the enforced payers and non-payers felt victimised and had rejected the obligation to pay. They tended to prioritise their own needs above those of their children partly as a result of poor economic circumstances, but this was also related to it not being the right time in their lives to pay. They therefore selected the mothers (and boyfriends/ husbands) as having the primary obligation to provide financial support for their non-resident children, especially if they believed they were better off financially. But it was argued that one of the principal reasons for rejecting the maintenance obligation was the failure of mothers to reciprocate with contact. This engendered powerful feelings of unfairness and injustice, which were exemplified in their demonising mothers through the construction of atrocity stories about their behaviour, and this confirmed their belief that any maintenance paid would simply be squandered. As Finch (1989) points out:

> Obligation, duty and responsibility, as understood in this sense [as products of negotiation], are commitments developed between real people, not abstract principles associated with particular kin relationships.

> (Finch, 1989: 181)

The *real* people with whom these fathers were developing commitments to pay maintenance were the mothers and not the children. This helps explain why the same man will pay maintenance willingly in one past relationship and refuse to pay in another. That was the situation for Malcolm and Harold, the respondents with two past relationships. Both of these fathers described the mothers of their second children as friends, whereas they despised the mothers of their children from their first past relationships. This 'friendship' with the mothers from their second past relationships enabled both fathers to put these second children 'first' when it came to financial obligations. This does not mean that these two fathers, or the others in this study, necessarily entered into explicit negotiations with the mothers about whether to pay maintenance or about how much to pay – though Harold did bargain with the first mother over his obligation. He was the only one, however, who used this approach, though the others may well have had explicit discussions in another forum with solicitors and the courts. The point is that the process of negotiation arises out of fathers' interactions with mothers both on an explicit and implicit level (Finch and Mason, 1993: 61).

The more implicit elements if this interaction are described by Finch and Mason (1993) as taking place when these normative guidelines are used to decide if the claim for support is legitimate. That is, people decide through a process of negotiation if the need for support and their individual capacity to give it are legitimate (Finch, 1989; Finch and Mason, 1993). Deciding upon the legitimacy of an obligation does not necessarily occur in explicit discussions between the interested parties. Rather, the normative guidelines highlight some of the more implicit thought processes that people engage in while deciding whether an obligation exists in the first instance, and whether it should be ongoing. Finch and Mason (1993) point out that the more implicit aspects of negotiation are exposed in the ways people try to legitimise their excuses for not giving support of the kind expected. 'Legitimate excuses' exist where people tend to give pre-eminence to the emotional aspects of the relationship over the financial need for support. Here we see how the 'excuses' provided by the enforced payers and non-payers for their reluctance to pay played down the economic importance of maintenance. The children in these relationships were deemed as not having a 'real' need for financial support, at least not in comparison with the fathers' own financial needs, or, as was demonstrated so clearly by Robert, not as important as the father's own emotional needs to have contact with his child. Here the fathers' desires for an ongoing relationship with their children took pre-eminence over their financial capacity to pay maintenance, as the continued commitment of the willing payers in the face of financial difficulties demonstrated. Yet the mother as the resident parent is the gatekeeper to the father's physical contact with children, thus her central position, between father and child, is fundamental for a relationship with children in the context of non–residency (Simpson *et al.*, 1995; Neale and Smart, 1997).

Central position of mothers

The centrality of the mother's position and its predominant importance in financial support are exposed through the guideline of balanced reciprocity. Fathers expected their parental relationship with mothers to be kept in balance. This expectation became most explicit when it was not fulfilled. Thus where the fathers perceived that the mothers were obstructing relationships with children, they said they would not get anything 'back in return' for maintenance. Contact and maintenance were therefore linked through the process of balanced reciprocity. This

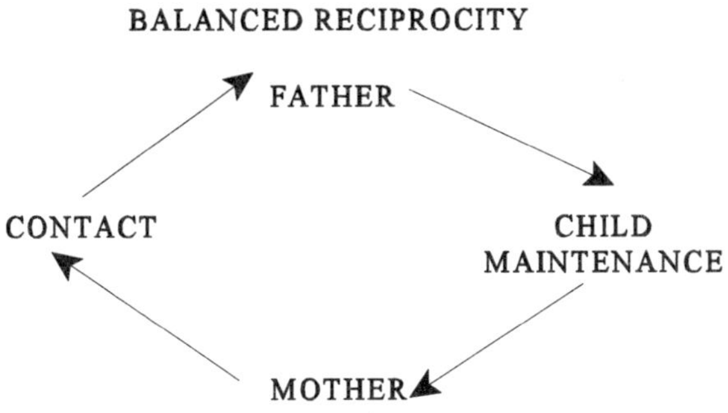

BALANCED RECIPROCITY

Figure 12.1 Reciprocal loop between contact and maintenance

guideline is more typical in adult relationships where people are expected to reciprocate fairly immediately by offering something back for support received (Finch and Mason, 1993: 146). The reciprocal loop between contact and maintenance is illustrated above in Figure 12.1.

When contact was desired but was not forthcoming, this signified a breakdown in reciprocal relations and it was extremely difficult to accept the obligation to pay maintenance within this context. Only Matthew, the one willing payer without contact, managed to override this.

Matthew expected nothing in return for maintenance; it was his expression of fatherly love and a duty owed to the mother. Thus he conflated his obligations to both the mother and the child and in doing so he applied a different guideline of reciprocity – generalised reciprocity to both these relationships. Generalised reciprocity is more typical in adult–child relationships; there is no expectation of an immediate return, as it forms part of the pattern of intergenerational exchange within families. Matthew was able to tolerate the imbalance in the parental relationship because he applied this guideline to his relationship with the mother as well as the child. However, his tolerance was also enhanced by the feelings of guilt he carried about the history of his relationship with both the mother and his son.

None of the enforced payers and non-payers carried such a powerful sense of guilt over the history of their failed relationships – rather they felt themselves to be victims at the mercy of pernicious mothers. This was clearly demonstrated by the construction of atrocity stories about mothers. Importantly, these stories illuminated how the legitimacy of the mother's claim for maintenance on behalf of children was rejected. The mother's conduct, specifically her perceived lack of support over the father's emotional relationships with children, was atrocious and beyond understanding. This exposes a second product of negotiations: the creation of understandings. The process of negotiation not only involves making a commitment to give material support but also involves reaching a shared understanding about what each party expects of the other (Finch, 1989). Therefore in deciding about the legitimacy of the 'need' for maintenance, the fathers were also deciding upon their 'willingness' to pay, based upon their own conduct and upon the conduct of the mother. Yet at the level of principle, all the men in this study agreed that fathers should pay maintenance. Given this, it is better to view the maintenance obligation as one that was found to be more or less acceptable, rather than suggest that the obligation in principle was ever seen as illegitimate. Additionally the fathers' (and mothers') circumstances altered over time and these changes had to be 'weighed up' to reassess the acceptability of this obligation. Finding the obligation either acceptable or unacceptable is therefore not fixed and is best represented as a continuum in which the strength of various contingent factors varies over time. The contingent factors highlighted by these respondents include the following:

Contingent factors related to capacity to pay
Fathers' income
Fathers' commitments to new second families
Mothers' socio-economic circumstances
Children's need for support
Past financial settlements

Contingent factors related to willingness to pay
History of relationship with mother and child(ren)
   how child conceived
   confidence over paternity
   length and quality of parental relationship
   length and quality of relationship with child (related to child's age)
   how relationships ended: blame/guilt
Parental relations post-separation
   reciprocal behaviour
   reaching shared understandings
   sharing parental responsibilities
   blame/guilt
Relations with child post-separation
   wanting and seeking contact
   having active contact
   guilt over reduced/unsatisfactory fatherhood role
Legal expectations and the threat of enforcement

Maintenance as a negotiated commitment

In reality, therefore, it depended upon circumstances whether maintenance was paid or not. Where payments were not enforced, they were the products of negotiated commitments emerging from the fathers' interactions with mothers and children. Yet because of the cross-cutting nature of legal enforcement, it was not possible to tell from the act of payment alone whether the fathers found this obligation acceptable. Legal enforcement curtailed the process of negotiation and was effective in making some of these fathers pay. But as Robert's case highlights, this could have long-lasting repercussions. Robert railed against the injustice of enforcement when he could not have contact with his son. Therefore, the maintenance obligation was negotiated, it was not viewed as an unconditional moral obligation owed to children on the sole basis of the biological father–child relationship, even though the fathers agreed that in principle they 'should pay'. The analysis of the enforced payers and non-payers indicates that these men did not fully accept a financial responsibility to provide for their children. It is more difficult to be sure about the payers. Although they demonstrated some sense of duty to financially provide, this was generally, though not exclusively, within the context of active relationships and defining themselves as having some capacity to pay. The question that cannot be definitively answered is, if the willing payers found themselves in similar circumstances to the enforced payers and non-payers would they express the same level of financial commitment to pay maintenance? Perhaps not.

So far the discussion has compared the willing payers with the enforced payers and non-payers together. This has highlighted how and in what ways the obligation of maintenance was a negotiated commitment and how the enforced payers and non-payers had rejected this obligation. But this raises a number of other questions – does this mean that enforced payers and non-payers have no sense of financial obligation to these children whatsoever? Or if they do, then how do they reconcile this sense of obligation when they do not pay? To answer these questions the enforced payers and non-payers need to be compared with one another.

COMPARING ENFORCED PAYERS AND NON-PAYERS

What became immediately apparent when comparing the two groups was that the non-payers faced a moral dilemma about their lack of financial support. This was the key difference between enforced payers and non-payers. Because the four enforced payers were actually paying maintenance (and Paul was also saving money for his child), albeit grudgingly, they did not face any dilemma about having rejected the maintenance obligation. This dilemma is worth exploring in more detail, as it highlights the complexity facing fathers in deciding what to do about their financial obligations within the context of non-residency.

The moral dilemma of maintenance

The moral dilemma of maintenance is explained as follows: On the one hand, the fathers who were not paying maintenance but wanted a relationship with their children (five in the seven non-paying relationships, excluding Harold who did not want contact and Alex who was unsure about his paternity) did feel some moral obligation to provide financial support for their children. They acknowledged that the children had a right to expect support from them and indeed they wanted to be in a position to 'give things' to them. On the other hand, they had rejected the maintenance obligation because they felt the mother had denied them contact. However, they also wanted to pay maintenance on the basis of generalised reciprocity with their children. Hence the concerns among non-payers about how the maintenance would be spent.

If the maintenance was spent 'inappropriately' by mothers, maintenance payments would not form part of intergenerational exchanges between father and child and, worse still, would further imbalance the exchange relationship of the parents. There was little point in paying, as fathers would not – or could not – trust mothers to spend it on the children, nor could they *see* for themselves, in the absence of contact, that the children were benefiting from payments, nor would the children know that their fathers were supporting them financially. Thus these men came to believe that maintenance payments would be squandered. To avoid this squandering of maintenance, all of the five non-payers who wanted contact with their children said the 'only way' they would provide financially was to save money in bank accounts for children or to 'give things' directly to the children themselves. In this way they could bypass the mother completely. This was how they attempted to reconcile their moral dilemma, as all financial provision could now operate upon the basis of generalised reciprocity between father and child. For these fathers there was therefore a tension between the guidelines of balanced and generalised reciprocity. They had to make a choice between basing their maintenance obligation on their relationships with children or on their relationships with mothers. Making a choice between these two guidelines was important, as the meanings underlying payments would differ substantially depending on which one was chosen as the basis for forming a commitment to pay. For example, the question these fathers might ask themselves is whether paying maintenance would primarily benefit the child or the mother? If they felt payment primarily favoured the mother, they were reluctant to pay and suggested that instead they would give 'things' or 'money' to the children themselves, or save money for them (Paul, the one enforced payer who was concerned about how the maintenance was spent, had saved money for his child, which would be realisable upon his death). One would therefore expect that these five non-payers were providing informal support. Not so: only one, Barry, gave clothing and saved money in a bank account for his children. Therefore it is argued that operating the guideline of generalised reciprocity, in a way that justifies non-payment of maintenance, is a means through which these fathers were constructing 'legitimate excuses' for their non-payment.

Legitimate excuses

Making their intentions to provide informal support explicit to an outside audience (such as the interviewer), but not actually doing so, was a way of sustaining these men's moral reputations as caring fathers. For the whole point of 'legitimate excuses' is to give an account of your action for *not* providing support in such a way that your moral reputation is maintained (Finch, 1989; Finch and Mason, 1993). This does not mean that excuses for not paying maintenance were illegitimate *per se*; but the conditions surrounding the giving of things or money directly to children necessitate actual contact with them (except if money was left as an inheritance). Otherwise, like maintenance payments, fathers would be dependent on mothers to pass items on and presumably the same feelings of mistrust of mothers would also apply to these items of informal support. This was how Barry felt about his informal support: he accused the mother of hiding or selling the clothes that he sent for the children. However, he was able to give other things (pocket money and treats) directly to his children, as he had physical contact with them. The intention to save money for children, however, served a more specific purpose.

Generosity and reciprocity

If the fathers did manage to give money from savings when the children were older, then this would enable fathers to appear generous in the eyes of the children themselves. This has implications for the father–child relationship in the longer term. For example on receipt of this gift, children might feel beholden to their fathers and respond by establishing contact independently of the mother. Thus giving a lump sum of money to children may help 'kick start' active relationships in the future. Whatever the intentions embedded within saving money, it exemplifies how those fathers in the non-paying relationships who had suggested this approach had *postponed* their relations with children till some future time. This postponement of relationships with children concurs with the findings of Simpson *et al.* (1995) in their study of divorced fathers. However, it also demonstrates how the fathers wanted to use money to aid their relationships with their children and it signifies how they had disengaged from explicit and direct negotiations with mothers, as they had unilaterally decided what their financial obligations were. In the absence of contact with children, these fathers had transformed the obligation to pay maintenance into one of giving informal support instead. In their minds at least, these men had not completely abandoned or dismissed their financial obligations as fathers. Nor had they given up all hope of having a relationship with their children when older.

The responses of the non-payers to their moral dilemma highlights how the central position of mothers (as the recipients of maintenance) created difficulties in translating financial obligations into practice. Fathers had to decide what guideline of reciprocity should underpin their payments – balanced or generalised reciprocity. Making a choice between these two guidelines was important, because the meanings underlying payments would differ substantially depending upon which one was seen as the main operational guideline on which to base a commitment to pay maintenance. The tension between these two guidelines of reciprocity was exemplified most clearly in some of the willing paying relationships, rather than in the non-paying relationships, because the latter were not paying maintenance and therefore not living with this tension. One case Stephen, is used to show how the different meanings applied to financial support elucidate the tension between the two guidelines of reciprocity in respect of child maintenance payments.

THE TENSION BETWEEN BALANCED AND GENERALISED RECIPROCITY

Stephen

Stephen was the most involved of all the fathers, in this sample, in his relationship with his child; his son came to stay with him every weekend and he saw him frequently during the week. Stephen and the mother got on well and they had both explicitly agreed to be fair to one another and 'give and take' in negotiations about their son. Stephen described how they both had 'given in' in equal measure over different parenting issues. This 'giving in' was indicative of balanced reciprocal relations. Yet even in this most ideal of situations, Stephen experienced difficulties in reconciling the tension between generalised and balanced reciprocity. This was evident in the ways Stephen had earmarked his maintenance payments.

Earmarking maintenance

Stephen had earmarked part of his maintenance payments for the exclusive use of his child. In his own mind he said he split the maintenance into an amount for 'board and lodging' and the remainder for 'clothes and shoes and things like that'. He also gave informal support by paying for school trips and hobbies and he gave his son pocket money. Because Stephen had earmarked part of the maintenance for his son's sole use (clothes and shoes), he was not entirely satisfied with his payments. He said he wanted to 'see what he was getting for his money'. For example, Stephen complained that when his son came to visit him and he was wearing new clothes or shoes, Stephen never knew if he had paid for all of it, part of it or none of it. In this way he couldn't *see* what was happening to the maintenance money and consequently he wanted to know how it was spent. Thus the maintenance money had been rendered *invisible* to Stephen. It was this invisibility that was problematic.

The invisibility of maintenance

Stephen described the invisibility of maintenance by contrasting the monies given for maintenance with Christmas and birthday presents. These forms of support were visible because his son knew that his father gave these gifts and he could acknowledge this by thanking his father. Stephen said this made him 'feel good'. In contrast, Stephen likened maintenance payments to the experience of using a credit card; it was like using a credit card because no 'feelings' were attached to this form of financial support. He described it thus:

> I suppose it's like when you're buying things on a Visa you don't see any money handed over you just sign away and you just get your goods and you go away don't you . . . and I think that that is the same feeling that you, you've got no benefit – you don't see

any – there is no feeling at all – or there is nothing there to say that you contributed towards paying for that . . .

The feelings Stephen could not enunciate were those of *intimacy*. Giving gifts is a distinguishing characteristic of intimate relationships. It is one way in which intimacy is maintained and thereby emotions and financial transactions are deeply interconnected (Cheal, 1987). Giftgiving is a means through which fathers can express their love, care and affection. It seems that giving money for child maintenance is unsatisfactory because the giver and receiver are not visible to one another. This is in part because money itself is a poor gift, as it can remove all traces of the person on whom the social relationship depends (Zelizer, 1994). As Stephen's case highlights, the invisibility of child maintenance operated to disconnect him from the meanings attached to giving this money.

There was an additional problem, however. Stephen's disconnection was made worse because it appeared that the mother – rather than Stephen – was giving these things to the son:

> but he just takes it for granted that his new clothes his mum's bought em . . .

> and I would like him to come and say 'look you know this is what me mum's bought this month' or 'she's going to get me this this month when she gets money from you' and things like that, and I don't really expect him to mention it but I would like his mum to have said something.

The utility of the money to express love and care was inadvertently transferred to the mother. The exchange was not money, nor was it the value of the money in pounds and pence, but the value it carried in *aiding intimacy* and demonstrating Stephen's love and care for his child. These symbolic meanings attached to maintenance were completely lost if it disappeared into household expenses, or if the mother retained the power to spend all the available resources provided by the father. The symbolic meaning of the money is being transferred to the mother. Once in her hands, she potentially gains this hidden utility at the father's expense. This highlights how Stephen's desire to 'know how maintenance was spent' was about enabling his status as giver to become visible to his child.

Herein lies the tension between the two guidelines of reciprocity, as payments made under each guideline corresponded to a different relationship and therefore had different meanings attached. Maintenance payments were problematic because the giver of the money was rendered invisible to the intended recipient – father to child. Thereby the meanings attached to the act of giving were also rendered invisible.

THE SYMBOLIC MEANING OF MAINTENANCE

The tension between generalised and balanced reciprocity – and therefore the particular problem of maintenance – resides in the different meanings fathers attach to their financial support. For as Zelizer (1996) explains:

> Monetary payments fall into three categories: gifts, entitlement, and compensation. Each one corresponds to a significantly different set of social relations and systems of meanings. People making payments use a number of earmarking techniques to distinguish those categories of social relations and meanings from each other, impose substantial controls over the proper uses of money received within each category, and attach great importance to the distinctions involved . . .
>
> (p. 481)

Earmarking money is a social process through which different symbolic meanings are attached to otherwise indistinct monies. This explains how fathers differentiated between maintenance and informal support. Informal support was earmarked for children only and thereby fell into the category of gift-giving. It corresponded directly with the father–child relationship and the principle of generalised reciprocity underpinning it. Informal support was relatively unproblematic; it was always given directly from father to child and thus it guaranteed that the father's status as giver was rendered visible. Given this, it is easy to see why those enforced payers and non-payers who had mistrustful relations with mothers wanted to give informal support instead of maintenance. This would be the 'only way' they could guarantee that, first, their status as giver was rendered visible and, second, the money given would be spent only on children. The meanings of love and care that they wanted to convey through financial provision would therefore be transmitted to children directly. The importance of informal support to convey messages of love was described explicitly by one of the non-payers. Ian said that he would like to give his daughter 'things' so that she would know that he was there for her, that he existed. It was not the material value of the items or gifts, but their value in conveying

Ian's feelings to his child. For, Ian said, there was 'no one in the world that could tell her he loved her'.

The importance of trust

The power of maintenance payments to transmit this message was diminished if it was to be paid against a backdrop of mistrust and failed reciprocal relations with mothers. The majority of non-payers and one enforced payer believed maintenance payments would only be squandered. They could not use maintenance to aid intimate relations with children or even gain contact with them. Moreover, it would be squandered because mothers (and perhaps stepfathers) could use this money to aid their own intimate relations with children or, worse, spend the money on themselves. Thus trust in mothers to spend maintenance on the children was fundamental to the expression of the fathers' care through financial provision. The importance of trust was demonstrated by the non-payers through their atrocity stories about mothers. The construction of these stories becomes explicable if they are related to more general gift-giving behaviour.

Imagine the responses of people if money given as a gift to a close relative, to help them out of financial difficulties, was spent on something frivolous like a holiday. How might they feel as a result? It is likely that they would not want to give monetary support in the future. Or if they felt obliged to continue to offer help, they may be more explicit about how the money should be used. Or they may even attempt to control the spending of this money by buying specific items instead. In equivalent terms, this is how some fathers in the enforced payment and non-payment groups wanted to behave in regard to maintenance. They preferred to provide financially through informal support. In that way they specifically earmarked informal support as a *gift*, and not maintenance. It also shows how money, in the form of savings, could be used to aid father–child relationships in the future. For giving gifts implies a long-term relationship (Zelizer, 1994).

Nonetheless, only one of the non-payers actually gave informal support. Therefore it was argued that transforming the obligation to pay maintenance into informal support acted as a legitimate excuse for not paying maintenance. Excuse or not, it is more complex than merely squirming out of a financial obligation. It also shows how relations with children were postponed, how the mother was bypassed, and how the process of negotiation was curtailed. In other words, these fathers were beginning to disengage, or had already become disengaged from involvement in their children's lives, albeit generally not through their own choosing. The majority of fathers without contact exhibited a deep need to interact with their children. They wanted to 'give' to their children, be with them and make them happy, be there for them when they were not physically with them, protect them, love them, help them, and support them in times of need. How could they manage all this within the context of having no or minimal involvement in their children's lives? There were at the very least limited outlets for the expression of such feelings or indeed no outlet in the absence of contact. Such feelings did find an outlet through the creation of 'good intentions' to provide informal support instead of maintenance. This highlights the importance of money in aiding fathers' relations with their children.

The usefulness of maintenance

Where fathers wanted continuing relations with children, they all wanted to use money directly, or indirectly, to convey their feelings of love 'for' or 'to' their children. For example, where maintenance was paid willingly it was given:

- as compensation for past failings in relations with mothers and children;
- as a substitute for not 'being there' for children on a frequent enough basis;
- to ease parental relations and act as a guarantee for contact – thus it acted as a manipulative tool in negotiations with mothers;
- in recognition of the child's entitlement;
- in recognition of the mother's entitlement as the primary carer of children.

Thus maintenance payments fell into a number of different categories of meaning. They could be 'gift maintenance', 'compensatory maintenance', or 'entitled maintenance', or indeed a combination of all three. What is not known is how fathers used money and gifts to express their feelings when they were living with children, or whether their behaviour in this regard was a continuation of what went before. Nonetheless it is reasonable to assume that when resident, fathers did not run the risk of having their acts of giving rendered invisible. This was not the case when non-resident. Thus it is argued that the usefulness of monies in non-resident relations all hinged upon creating opportunities that would render the giver visible. Fathers could then convey their feelings for children within the act of giving itself. The most obvious way for fathers to render their status visible was to encourage mothers to enable contact. Hence the importance of maintenance as a tool in negotiations. Mothers could thereby earn their entitlement to claim maintenance on behalf of children. Thus entitled, maintenance could reflect the mothers' and children's entitlement simultaneously.

Whether fathers were manipulating mothers or not, it would seem that within willing paying relationships an understanding had been reached that parental relationships should be kept in balance. However, even in the absence of active relations, the mother could still play an important role as the recipient of the message that was underlying payment. That payment was a means of making amends for past failings. This was exemplified by Matthew, the one father who paid maintenance willingly in the absence of contact. In effect, his payments were simultaneously a *gift* and a *compensation*, as he expected nothing in return. Thus gift maintenance, entitled maintenance and compensatory maintenance were useful and meaningful to these fathers in their relationships with mothers and children. There was no need to transform the obligation of maintenance into informal support, as these fathers were in a position to give gifts directly to their children or endow part of their maintenance payments as 'gift maintenance'. Fathers were therefore willing to pay.

SUMMARY

The aim of this qualitative study was to try to understand why some fathers paid maintenance while others did not. To that end the twenty relationships of the eighteen fathers in this qualitative sample were categorised on two criteria – first by whether maintenance was paid and second by whether these payments were enforced. Three groups emerged: willing payers where maintenance was paid but not enforced, enforced payers and non-payers. From the comparisons made between the groups it became apparent that crucial to understanding how financial obligations operated in practice was the nature of fathers' social relations with mothers and children. It was within the context of these relationships that the fathers' commitments to pay maintenance (and to provide informal support) were created, sustained and sometimes dissolved. The interaction between social relations and financial obligations was exemplified in two main ways. First, through the process of negotiation and, second, through the process of earmarking money. Both of these perspectives helped illuminate the specific nature of non-resident fathers' financial obligations. In particular, they helped to expose the tension between the fathers' relationships with children and the fathers' relationships with mothers. This tension found expression within the different normative guidelines that operated within each set of relationships and in the different meanings that were applied to maintenance payments and informal support.

Spending money on informal support was an important aspect of non-resident fathers' social relations with children. Indeed this may have been a continuance of fathers' expressive relations with children when resident with them. But perhaps informal support took on greater importance in the context of non-residency, as it could aid intimate relations with children through the provision of gifts and treats, entertainment and holidays. It was primarily a medium through which fathers could express their feelings to their children directly. Therefore, strictly speaking, informal support was not a form of payment. It was not an obligation or a responsibility 'owed' to children, but was mainly an integral part of active relationships. Thus it was distinguished from maintenance.

Child maintenance was much more problematic. The fathers in this qualitative sample did indeed view it as an obligation 'owed' to children, but in reality, as maintenance payments were given to the mother, this obligation was open to negotiation. Not only did fathers have to negotiate directly with mothers over contact arrangements with regard to children, but they were also negotiating the acceptability of paying maintenance 'to' the mother. They were therefore deciding upon the legitimacy of her claim for maintenance on behalf of children. Her claim was viewed as legitimate if she at least enabled contact between the father and child. The expectation was that the parents' relationship should operate upon the basis of balanced reciprocity. The proper thing for the mother to do was to enable the father to have continuing contact and the proper thing for the father to do was to pay maintenance. Where the fathers perceived that the mother was obstructing contact, then her claim for maintenance was felt to be illegitimate. This was the main distinction between the groups.

All except one of the fathers in the willing group had contact with their children and they found their maintenance payments both useful and meaningful in their relationships. This underpinned their commitment to pay. First, payments could be used to 'ease', persuade or even coerce mothers into agreeing to contact arrangements. Second, maintenance could be earmarked in whole or in part as a gift, as compensation or as part of the mother's and/or child's entitlement. On the whole, the willing payers tended not to distinguish between gift maintenance, entitled maintenance and compensatory maintenance because the mother's claim for maintenance was viewed as legitimate. Thus she could receive it in her own right, either as compensation for bad conduct on the part of the father (adultery, for example) or as entitlement in her role as carer. Giving maintenance as a gift to the mother was rare because gifts are given with no expectation of a return and, as already highlighted, mothers were expected to reciprocate for maintenance received by enabling contact. It seemed that the one willing payer who had no contact with his child did pay gift maintenance. He expected nothing in return for maintenance, as he did not blame the mother entirely for his lack of contact, but in addition he described his maintenance as an expression of his fatherly love. Gift maintenance therefore tended to reflect the father–child relationship and not the mother–father relationship. The enforced payers and non-payers, however, did distinguish between these different types of payments.

The enforced payers and non-payers had all found the maintenance obligation unacceptable because they felt the mother's claim was illegitimate. They had either decided that the mother and children did not need it, or that the mother did not deserve it as she had obstructed contact, or that she could not be trusted to spend it only on the children. Maintenance payments would therefore be squandered; they could not be used as a means of manipulating the mother to agree to contact, nor would the children benefit from payment. Consequently, maintenance payments were both useless and meaningless to these men in their relationships. In response, they tended to earmark their actual payments (enforced payers) or intended payments (non-payers) as gift maintenance to be spent only on children. However, given the lack of trust in mothers expressed by some of these fathers (mainly among the non-payers), there was no means of ensuring that the children would receive this gift. They therefore refused to pay. This kind of tautological argument, however, worked as a legitimate excuse for the non-payment of maintenance. In effect, they were announcing to the world that if the circumstances through which the maintenance obligation could be realised were more acceptable to them, they would pay it.

Clearly the processes of negotiation and earmarking are closely related. They have helped to demonstrate not only what is involved in developing a commitment to pay maintenance, but also the peculiarities of maintenance as monies. The maintenance obligation was owed to children, but because the mothers were the actual recipients of these monies, it mattered very much how they were spent. Mothers were in effect acting as trustees – trustees of the fathers' relationship with their children and trustees of both the maintenance monies and the expressions of care attached to them. It is highly probable that where fathers had contact with their children, maintenance payments were not such an important medium for the expression of care directly 'to' children. Conversely, it seemed to be a very important medium for the fathers without contact, hence they earmarked it as gift maintenance. However, it was highly unsatisfactory in this regard, as essentially maintenance payments were invisible. The children would not necessarily know their fathers were paying it and the fathers would not know whether the children were benefiting from it. The non-payers in particular were therefore left with nothing but 'good intentions' to provide financially in other ways. Thus reciprocity and entitlement were inextricably linked. The child's right or entitlement to support from both parents depends on the ability of the parents to share and reciprocate over caring and financial responsibilities. Nonetheless, the reality was that some of these men were not providing any form of financial support for their children and the vital question for policy makers is how can they capture the 'good intentions' of non-payers to encourage commitments to pay maintenance?

13 Concluding discussion

We began this book by describing the way non-resident fathers had become vilified as feckless 'Deadbeat Dads' in some media and political discourse. Clearly there are some non-resident fathers who through anger, hurt or general vindictiveness are failing to support their children financially and in other ways, although they can afford to. But a much more pervasive picture that emerges from this research is that of men struggling to be the fathers of non-resident children.

What these men had to do was to surmount a number of internal and external problems when they became non-resident fathers. They had to deal with the practical difficulties of life – they had to provide money for their own household and their family; they had to provide adequate housing so that children had a place to visit; they had to have the time to spend with their children; and they needed energy and patience to be active parents. They also had to deal with the sense of loss over daily interactions with their children and had to adjust to parenting full-time on a part-time basis, if they mainly saw their children at weekends. Similarly, tensions could exist where the mother and father expected different codes of conduct and behaviour from their children in their respective households. These factors could have an impact on the fathers' relationships with their children.

In the first qualitative study we found that children and grandmothers (particularly the fathers' parents) were major actors in maintaining contact. The children of non-resident fathers have generally not been seen as significant actors who negotiate contact time with their fathers either directly or through their mothers. Some children in this sample were prepared to travel long distances on their own to see their fathers and some negotiated a change of residency across their parents' households. The age of children was important, not necessarily in terms of the continuity of contact (we had no evidence to explore this), but the nature of contact where it was already established. Some fathers found that as their children got older they were 'growing away from home' and following their own interests; others felt they had got closer to their children and saw them more frequently and on an individual basis. These variable outcomes might explain the results in the quantitative survey – that the older the age of the younger child, the greater the likelihood that fathers would *not* have regular contact. The fathers in the first qualitative study reported that their young teenage children were busy with employment, friends and other interests and that they (the fathers) had to learn to accept that they were taking second place. This of course may be just as much a feature of resident fatherhood as non-resident fatherhood. Importantly, these findings highlight the limitations in measuring non-resident fathers' relationships with children as if they were a single unit who had uniform contact arrangements. Grandmothers could also be intimately involved in maintaining contact with children, not only for their own relationships as grandparents but also acting as guardians for the fathers' relationships. More research is needed to find out not only how much support is offered by grandmothers, but also how this works in practice and under what circumstances.

There remains a debate about the importance of contact between non-resident fathers and their children. In contrast to the findings of Simpson *et al.* (1995), whose data were collected in 1991, we found that fathers were very keen to maintain contact with their children after relationship breakdown. It has previously been common to assume that it was in the best interests of all those involved to make a 'clean break', and for fathers to give up contact, especially where there was conflict with mothers. It was the received wisdom that by not seeing their children, the fathers made life easier for all concerned, and that by maintaining contact, the misery and heartache that occurred after the relationship breakdown continued indefinitely (Goldstein, Freud and Solnit, 1973). Research in the USA by Wallerstein and Kelly (1980) and in Britain by Richards and Dyson (1982) has since led to a revision of this view. It is now thought that it is better for children, if not for their parents, for the fathers to maintain contact, not only for the child's emotional health but also for its social and cognitive development (that is, where abuse is not a feature of the father–child relationship). The terms of the Children Act 1989 reflect this view that the sharing of parental responsibility should be encouraged – under this Act the old notion of 'care and control' or custody being awarded to one parent has been swept away. Rather it is hoped that parents will seek to make their own arrangements, with the law stepping in as a last resort to arrange the residency of children and contact. Nonetheless, the barriers presented by travelling large distances and long gaps in contact, find some men questioning whether the effort was 'worth it'. At the same time, however, though some fathers were resigned to loss of contact, others remain very bitter and angry and felt they had been let down by the legal system, which would not act to enforce contact effectively. As Walker (1996) has pointed out, it is difficult for any external authority to ensure contact, or at least not without risk of damage to all involved. Yet Smart and Neale (1997) argue that there has been a 'strong presumption' in favour of contact and that now judicial treatment has adopted a 'rigid and dogmatic' form which is harmful. Mothers are now viewed as being 'implacably hostile' when reluctant to allow contact, whereas before it was believed they were acting in the best interests of the children and in any case it was felt to be unrealistic to enforce it as it would necessitate separating out the interests of the child from the circumstances of the parent with daily primary care. Increasingly, argue Neale and Smart (1997), the legal profession is using coercive techniques including the threat of imprisonment – even in the face of evidence in some cases where the children were visibly distressed during supervised contact visits with their fathers – and where the previous behaviour of fathers, towards mothers at least, has been known to be violent. Under this egalitarian ethos Neale and Smart question 'whether it will soon be possible to be critical of any kind of fathering'.

What this serves to highlight is the interwoven nature of the needs and interests of mothers, children and non-resident fathers. Giving primacy to the needs of either of the parents can result in losing the best interests of children – a fine balance needs to be struck; yet the needs and interests of these three major parties may constantly shift, requiring a responsive and refined approach in the exercise of the law. We certainly do not advocate that all fathers should have contact with their children, but there must come a point where men's complaints about their lost relationships with their children must be taken seriously. Legal enforcement is not the answer, and in any event it comes too late after relationships between the parents have completely broken down. Mediation seems the most hopeful way forward, though it has been argued that this approach can also coerce mothers to comply with contact.

As we have seen, contact with the child is very closely associated with whether child support is paid. The Child Support Act 1991 was based on the principle that biological fathers have an absolute and unreserved responsibility to provide financial support for their children throughout their lives. Not all the fathers accepted this principle. The maintenance obligation is one that was negotiated. Fathers arrived at a commitment to pay maintenance by weighing up the strength of the financial obligation in the context of their own personal, financial and family circumstances and those of the mother and children. In practice, the obligation to pay was never unconditional, it always depended on circumstances. It partly depended on the father's ability to pay, the children's material need for maintenance and the mother's and her partner's (if she had a partner) ability to provide financially. But most importantly it was the history of the relationship with the mother that was the overriding factor in making a commitment to pay maintenance. From the fathers' perspective it was mothers who were claiming maintenance (albeit on behalf of children), not the children. This claim had to be *legitimised* before fathers would pay. Primarily, the mother's right to claim maintenance on behalf of children was accepted if she at least recognised, if not actively supported, the father's independent relationship with his child(ren). If the mothers failed to accept the father–child relationship or failed to sustain it through granting contact, then the fathers found this extremely difficult to comprehend. This incomprehension induced an overwhelming sense of victimisation and powerlessness among those men who wanted a relationship with their children but were unable to achieve it in the face of what they saw as selfish and callous mothers. The resultant attitude tended to be that there was no point in paying maintenance because the children would not know their fathers were supporting them, there was no guarantee that the money would be spent for the children's benefit and the fathers were 'paying for a child they were not seeing'. Thus not only would fathers get 'nothing back' in return for maintenance (contact with their children), but payment was meaningless because the fathers' act of giving was rendered invisible to the children themselves. Children would be unaware of the symbolic expression of love and care embedded within the act of giving maintenance money, particularly when, in the absence of contact, there was no other means through which fathers could demonstrate their affections to children directly. Therefore the obligation to pay maintenance was intimately linked with contact through the relationship with the mother, and the different outcomes of the process of negotiation (payment or non-payment) primarily hinged upon this relationship.

As we have seen, financial obligations are not straightforward; non-resident fathers are one step removed from their children and consequently it appears that money takes on greater significance in these relationships. Whether we like it or not, men seem to use money to at least ease relationships with mothers, if not to persuade mothers to agree to contact. Maintenance money is also earmarked for specific purposes and endowed with particular meanings. The maintenance obligation therefore is not just a bill to be paid, but is given on the basis of the nature of the relationships that underpin it. Thus we have different expressions of the obligation – gift maintenance, entitled maintenance and compensatory maintenance. For some, maintenance was enforced and enforced maintenance carried no endowed meaning other than through its withdrawal, which could send messages to the mother of the father's disquiet and anger.

Child support, not contact, has been the most salient and controversial policy arena concerning non-resident fathers in recent years and the approach to child support obligations has been transformed in a very short period. Under the French Code Napoleon of 1804, 'The search for paternity is forbidden' (section 340). In British case law and in practice if not in statute, by the end of the 1980s the rights of non-resident fathers to have control over and access to their children had become dissipated. Their obligations to maintain their former partner and children had effectively lapsed as well. The approach to financial responsibility for children tended to be based on the household formation – or social relationships – whether they were biological or not. Thus stepfathers took on the financial responsibility for children in their care when they were recognised as a 'child of the family'. In practice, social fathering rather than biological fathering had become the accepted basis on which a child–father relationship existed and financial obligations were determined. As Maclean (1993) notes, in the private law in the United Kingdom the apportionment of financial responsibility between social parenthood and biological parenthood tended to be pragmatic and based on the needs and resources of all involved rather than upon any firm rule.

However, at the end of the 1980s a combination of factors led to a remarkable reassertion of the obligations of biological fathers and separated partners to each other. It arose in the legal context of burgeoning recognition of children's rights as capable individuals – which began with the Matrimonial and Family Proceedings Act 1984 where courts were instructed to give primacy to the interests of children when settling divorce. It partly arose in the political context of 'moral panic' associated with the Victorian values/'back to basics' anxieties of the Conservative Governments of Margaret Thatcher and John Major. The practice of the legal profession to make low child maintenance awards to protect lone parents' full entitlement to social assistance (Eekelaar, 1991), and the failure of the DSS liable relative sections to actively pursue maintenance from parents, were said to be deeply embarrassing to the Conservative Government under Margaret Thatcher, which was committed to encouraging individual responsibility and reducing the welfare role of the state (Maclean, 1994). It was also partly generated by anxiety about the rising level of public expenditure associated with the increase in lone parents and their increased dependency on social assistance and public housing. It was certainly reinforced by anxieties about the impact of family breakdown on the living standards of lone parent families and the impact of this poverty, and the disruption and the experience of living in a lone parent household, on the well-being and future development of children (Rodgers and Prior, 1998).

Though not all the legislation affecting family law in recent years has been influenced by all these factors, one or more of the factors have been influential in determining the nature of the Children Act 1989, which affirmed that in care proceedings following separation and divorce the best interest of the child should be 'paramount'; the Child Support Act 1991 established an absolute obligation of non-resident fathers to provide financial support for their biological children throughout their lives; the Family Law Act 1996, as well as seeking to remove the vestiges of fault in divorce proceedings, will establish a 'framework' for information giving and mediation in marital breakdown. There is more legislation expected including an Act to cover pension splitting on divorce, legislation to establish the rights of unmarried fathers and a major reform of the child support system.

We have discussed the problems with the present child support scheme in the introduction to Chapter 8. At the time of writing, the Government are consulting on a Green Paper (UK, Cmnd 3992, 1998) that will substantially reform the existing scheme.

It was a grave error to seek to establish a child support regime based on a rigid (and yet complicated) formula administered by the DSS. This area of policy calls for a degree of flexible, individualised justice that probably cannot be handled within the disciplines and culture of social security. When the CSA was being planned, it might have been wiser and more effective to have reformed the existing court arrangements to increase consistency of adjudication, and to establish mechanisms for better review and enforcement.

What we have now is a split system for child support – the DSS dealing almost exclusively with benefit cases, while non-benefit cases make private arrangements between the parents themselves or with the support of solicitors. At the same time the Lord Chancellor's Department under the Family Law Act 1996 is experimenting with an information service and a mediation service following marital breakdown (but not cohabitation breakdown) covering the arrangements for children, the distribution of property and other assets – in fact everything except child support. The Family Law Act has not yet been implemented and the decision to reform child support could have presented an opportunity for thrashing out a common strategy and more coherent set of arrangements for negotiating contact, child support and other matters consequent on the breakdown of relationships when children are involved. The difficulty is that we are not starting from scratch – the Child Support Agency exists; the Family Law Act exists, after a torrid passage through Parliament. The Lord Chancellor does not want to go back to the drawing board and certainly is reluctant to take on the poisoned chalice of child support, so we are left after the reforms with a set of incoherent arrangements. This is despite the vague promises in the new child support proposals of having an 'active family policy'.

Though the proposed reforms have many laudable improvements, including a disregard in Income Support, the weakness of the proposed new scheme for child support is that the assessments are still formula-driven and still imposed and enforced completely independently of negotiations between the parents about other arrangements for financial support, contact and other related matters. The results of this research show that no child support scheme has a prospect of success unless it is based on negotiation between the parents, which is recognised as fair, and the perception of fairness on the fathers' part depends more than anything on their ability (and the former partners' willingness) to have shared parental responsibility for their children. The mistake that the Child Support Act made was that the state took a robust moral stance in the interests of the taxpayer and imposed a law on people who, it has been demonstrated, were not prepared to consent to it. What is needed is a service that enables these fathers and mothers to work out arrangements for child support, contact and other matters that concern them. Of course the state and taxpayers have an interest and that interest can be represented by a framework of guidelines, even a formula, but only if it is able to take account of exceptional cases and individual circumstances in a reasonably flexible manner. It is possible that the tribunal system proposed in the Green Paper could become the vehicle for providing such a degree of flexibility if it is allowed to operate fairly and freely and is not circumscribed by statute. However, it ought to be possible for the adjudication elements to be returned to a reformed family court system with the collection and enforcement remaining the responsibility of a successor to the Child Support Agency.

From time to time the Green Paper recognises the need for children to have clear signals that their father cares for them and is paying maintenance (see for example Chapter 18, para 3). We have found that this is a critical issue. At the moment, in the majority of cases the father is paying informal support and that is recognised by the child because for the most part it is given directly to the child. If the formal child support regime is going to become more effective, then informal support is likely to diminish. Children are going to think that their fathers' contribution (and care) for them is less and this is going to affect their relationships with their fathers. The issue of the salience and transparency of child support is a major grievance of fathers, an important reason for not paying and a cause of non-compliance. Fathers (resident and non-resident) very commonly define their role and express their affection and commitment through the breadwinner role. When they are non-resident and do not have contact, they do not see any recognition of their financial contribution and do not pay or pay informally. It would be in everyone's best interest for there to be a formal arrangement for informing children (over a certain age) that their fathers are contributing to their upkeep.

There is a proposal in the Green Paper to charge all fathers, regardless of their incomes and family commitments, a minimum child support of £5 per week. At present, fathers with new children to support and who are on Income Support or have a low income are excused paying any child support. The justification for this proposal is that personal circumstances cannot negate responsibility for one's children. But this 'principle' competes with the principle that Income Support is supposed to be a floor, a safety net. Although that principle has already been breached by direct deductions for utility debts and Social Fund loans, it is a further unfortunate undermining of the safety net. It is also effectively a transfer from one poor family to another possibly poor family. Indeed, what it does for lone mothers on Income Support is just about compensate them for the abolition of the lone parent premium in Income Support – by cutting the Income Support of their former partners. There is a balance to be struck between parents and the taxpayer. The taxpayer takes primary responsibility for supporting the children of those parents who are not in the labour market, and has, and will continue to have, responsibility for supporting the children of lone mothers on Income Support. This has been the collective arrangement considered reasonable since 1948. It is an understandable aspiration to get fathers to contribute what they can, where they can, but not where they cannot and there is a risk that other children will suffer.

Connected to this is the fact that there is no limit to the maximum maintenance that non-resident fathers will be expected to pay. Judging from our results, there will be serious opposition from better-off fathers if the scheme expects them to pay more than the costs of a child and anything more than necessary to lift their children beyond the scope of the benefits system. Why should the state determine how much fathers should pay for their non-resident child when it does not involve the taxpayer? It would be considered an intolerable assault on personal liberty if it happened in a couple family.

This is perhaps an example of the hint of residual moral vilification of non-resident fathers that still emerges from time to time in the Green Paper. In general, the language of the Green Paper is a great improvement on that of 'Children Come First'. For example, the Green Paper follows our usage of non-resident fathers instead of absent fathers. However, in Chapter One, para. 1 we are told that child support will be 'firmly enforced' – *effectively* enforced might have been received better by citizens experiencing government intervention in the complexities and intimacies of their private lives. Later in Chapter Two paras 25 and 26 there is the assumption that all fathers leave their children. Again we hear the echoes of the 'walking away' language of Mrs Thatcher, which so disastrously inspired the Child Support Acts. Our research shows that some fathers are never given a chance to live with their children. In other cases mothers take their children and leave the father. Generally, separation occurs after much unhappiness. In the end, parents leave each other by mutual agreement. Many fathers are sad and frustrated at not being able to see their children as much or as often as they would like. Their lives, like their children's and former partner's, have been disrupted. They are much more likely to be out of employment and dependent on a low income. Nevertheless, the majority are in touch with their children and the majority are paying either formal or informal support. If policy is to be successful in helping parents, both parents, to care for their children, it needs to build on these positive elements in these human relationships.

According to Smart (1997) there has been, in the debates about the decline and destabilisation of the family, a wishful thinking where it is hoped to return 'the family' to some idealised state unaffected by social change. However, what appears not to have changed is that fathers are still keen to point out that they do care about their non-resident children – and that is the problem! Rather convolutedly, it is because they care about maintaining their role as fathers and because they continue to want a close, intimate and fulfilling relationship with their children, that they can become reluctant to pay maintenance. The majority want to fulfil all their parental obligations, social, emotional and financial, but it seems that one is unsatisfactory without the others. There is therefore in some sense no need to 'reinforce' parental obligations – they exist and are accepted already. But there is a need to facilitate them through an increased understanding of the emotional and moral turmoil that follows in the wake of family separation or in the wake of cohabitation breakdown or non-marital births.

Notes

1 For example, a cartoon in the *Sunday Times* published on 11 July 1993 depicted a pregnant mother in a wedding dress, with three other children poking their heads out from under her dress, arm in arm with her bridegroom, who is an official from the Department of Social Security, while in the background the non-resident father with an enormous belly and 'free love' tattooed on his arm swills beer. The caption reads 'Sugar Daddy!'

2 The National Survey of Families and Households (NFSH) based at the University of Wisconsin–Madison (Seltzer, 1991; Sweet and Bumpass, 1987); and the National Survey of Children, begun in 1976 in Pennsylvania, which examined the development of changing family forms and the role of non-resident fathers (Furstenberg, 1988b; Furstenberg and Nord, 1985; Furstenberg, Nord, Petersen and Zill, 1983). The survey of Income and Programme Participation has also been used to study non-resident fathers (Sorenson, 1997).

3 Marsh's study has never been published, but it is interesting that he found that the non-resident fathers in the NCDS claimed to have a much higher level of contact with their children than Bradshaw and Millar (1991) had found when asking lone mothers. The proportion of divorced men having contact with their children was 81 per cent and for separated men it was 90 per cent.

4 The respondents to the FWLS are asked 'How many children, if any, do you have who do NOT live here? Please include step children and those who have set up their own homes.' Those with any such children are then asked 'How many of these children who do not live here with you fall into the following groups? Over 18, 16–18, 11–15, 5–10, 3–4, 0–2?' This is a slightly different definition from the one used to define non-resident fathers in our study, in that it includes non-natural children of the father and the upper age limit is 18 rather than in our study 16–18 if in full-time education. We also required that they lived with their mothers.

5 There was some difficulty combining the income data, which NOP and OPCS recorded using different banding systems. It was possible to combine the data from the two omnibus surveys using a crude banding of low, below £10,000 per year; medium, £10,000–£20,000; and high, over £20,000.

6 Income was excluded from the regression because of the number of cases with missing data.

7 We also tried weighting using the coefficients from the logistic regression, but it made no difference to the outcome.

8 There were twenty cases who were 'missing' for either social class or marital status. The weights for these were set to 1.0. Of these, fifteen had been interviewed and five had refused.

9 Or at least potentially a lone mother – some could have moved directly from their previous partnership to form this new one.

10 There is a debate about whether the appropriate comparison is with all fathers or men not living with children. Residential fathers have a higher employment rate than single men. Fathers have been chosen for comparison, because the sample are fathers and some of them live with children.

11 First adult = .61, spouse = .39, couple = 1.00, each child aged 16–18 = .36, 13–15 = .27, 11–12 = .25, 8–10 = .23, 5–7 = .21, 2–4 = .18, 0–1 = .09.

12 The threshold = £92 per week for equivalent net income, £89 per week for net income after child support, £92 per week net income after housing costs and £89 per week after housing costs, travel-to-work costs, child support and child-care costs.

13 This may not be a reliable indication of the prevalence of shared care. The screening question sought to identify men whose children normally lived with their mother in another household. Hence some shared care arrangements might have been missed.

14 Child support is used here and elsewhere as a generic term for all kinds of maintenance payments in respect of children and not just those arranged through the Child Support Agency. Maintenance is used interchangeably with child support.

15 Use of the CSA would only be a requirement in cases where the parent with care was on benefit. In cases where she was not on benefit, the parents would always have the option of reaching voluntary agreements. If they had made a settlement before the 1991 Act came into effect (April 1993), and the parent with care did not claim benefit, the voluntary agreement or court order would remain in place unless either parent chose to make an application to the CSA.

16 That is, children spend roughly equal amounts of time living in their mother's and father's households.

References and further reading

Abbott, D. (1996) 'The Child Support Act 1991: the lives of parents with care living in Liverpool', *Journal of Social Welfare and Family Law* 18(1): 21–36.

Ahrons, C.R. and Rodgers, R.H. (1987) *Divorced Families Meeting the Challenge of Divorce and Remarriage*, London: Norton.

Ahrons, C.R. and Wallisch, L.S. (1987) 'The relationship between former spouses', in D. Perlman and S. Duck (eds) *Intimate Relationships: Developments, Dynamics and Deterioration*, London: Sage.

Allan, G. and Skinner, C. (1991) *Handbook for Research Students in the Social Sciences*, London: Falmer Press.

Amato, P.R. (1996) 'Fathers' contributions to their children's lives: human, financial and social capital', Paper given to Australian Family Research Conference.

Amato, P.R. and Keith, B. (1991) 'Parental divorce and the well being of children: a meta analysis', *Psychological Bulletin* 110: 26–46.

Amato, P.R. and Rezac, S.J. (1994) 'Contact with non resident parents, interpersonal conflict, and children's behaviour', *Journal of Family Issues* 15(2): 191–207.

Ambrose, P., Harper, J. and Pemberton, R. (1983) *Surviving Divorce, Men beyond Marriage*, Brighton: Wheatsheaf.

Arendell, T. (1995) *Fathers and Divorce*, London: Sage.

Argyle, M. and Henderson, M. (1985) *The Anatomy of Relationships*, Harmondsworth: Penguin.

Augustus, P. (1995) *Baby Father 2*, London: The X Press.

Australian Institute of Family Studies (1992) *Family Matters* 32.

Australian Institute of Family Studies (1996) *Family Research: Pathways to Policy*, Conference Handbook, Brisbane: AIFS.

Backett, K.C. (1982) *Mothers and Fathers*, London: Macmillan.

Backett, K.C. (1987) 'The negotiation of fatherhood', in C. Lewis and M. O'Brien (eds) *Reassessing Fatherhood – New Observations on Fathers and the Modern World*, London: Sage.

Barber, D. (1975) *Unmarried Fathers*, London: Hutchinson.

Barker, R.W. (1994) *Lone Fathers and Masculinities*, Aldershot: Avebury.

Barnes, H. and Kilkey, M. (1997) *Children and Social Exclusion in Europe*, European Observatory Paper, Lisbon.

Bartfield, J. and Meyer, D.R. (1994) 'Are there really deadbeat dads?', *Social Science Review* 68(2): 219–35.

Becker, H.S. (1960) 'Notes on the concept of commitment', *American Journal of Sociology* 66: 32–40.

Beilharz, P. (1996) 'Cities and money – back to Berlin, via Chicago', in *Thesis Eleven* No. 46: 115–26.

Bennett, F. and Chapman, V. (1990) *The Poverty of Maintenance*, London: Child Poverty Action Group (CPAG).

Bertaux, D. and Delcroix, C. (1992) 'Where have all the Daddies gone?', in U. Bjornberg (ed.) *European Parenting in the 1990s: Contradictions and Comparisons*, New Brunswick and London: Transaction Publishers.

Bertoia, C. and Drakich, J. (1995) 'The fathers' rights movement: contradictions in theory and practice', in W. Marsiglio (ed.) *Fatherhood: Contemporary Theory, Research and Social Policy*, London: Sage.

BIB (1993) *Changing Families in Changing Societies*, Proceedings of the Brussels Conference, Wiesbaden: BIB.

Bjornberg, U. and Kollind, A.-K. (eds) (1996) *Men's Family Relations*, Stockholm: Almqvist and Wiksell.

Blain, J. (1993) 'The daily construction of fatherhood; men talk about their lives', in T. Haddad (ed.) *Men and Masculinities; A Critical Anthology*, Toronto: Canadian Scholars' Press.

Boden, F. and Childs, M. (1996) 'Paying for procreation: child support arrangements in the UK', *Feminist Legal Studies* 4(2): 131–57.

Bohannan, P. (1970) *Divorce and After*, New York: Doubleday.

Boleat, M. (1985) *Mortgage Payment Difficulties*, Building Societies Association.

Borrowdale, A. (1994) *Reconstructing Family Values*, London: SPCK.

Bott, E. (1957) *The Family and Social Networks*, London: Tavistock.

Bowlby, J. (1965) *Childcare and the Growth of Love*, Harmondsworth: Penguin.

Bowlby, J. (1980) *The Making and Breaking of Affectional Bonds*, London: Tavistock.

Bradshaw, J. (1994) 'What is wrong with the Child Support Act?', Parliamentary Brief.

Bradshaw, J. and Millar, J. (1991) *Lone Parent Families in the UK*, DSS Research Report No. 6, London: HMSO.

Bramley, G., Munro, M. and Lancaster, S. (1996) *Household Formation Literature Review*, London: Department of Education.

Brannen, J. (1992) 'British parenthood in the wake of the New Right: some contradictions and changes', in U. Bjornberg (ed.) *European Parenting in the 1990s*, New Brunswick and London: Transaction Publishers.

Brannen, J. and Moss, P. (1987) 'Fathers in dual earner households – through mothers' eyes', in C. Lewis and M. O'Brien (eds) *Reassessing Fatherhood: New Observations on Fathers and the Modern Family*, London: Sage.

Braver, S.H., Wolchik, S.A., Sandler, I.N., Fogas, B.S. and Zventina, D. (1991) 'Frequency of visitation by divorced fathers: differences in reports by fathers and mothers', *American Journal of Orthopsychiatry* 61: 448–54.

Bryman, A. (1992) *Quantity and Quality in Social Research*, London: Routledge.

Bryman, A., Byetheway, B., Allat, P. and Keil, T. (eds) (1987) *Rethinking the Life Cycle*, Basingstoke: Macmillan.

Buck, N. (1994) 'Housing and residential mobility', in N. Buck *et al.* (eds) *Changing Households: The British Households Panel Survey 1990–92*, ESRC Research Centre on Micro-Social Change, University of Essex.

Bull, J. (1993) *Housing Consequences of Relationship Breakdown*, London: HMSO.

Bull, J. and Stone, M. (1989) *Housing and Relationship Breakdown*, mimeo, York: Social Policy Research Unit.

Bumpass, L.L. and Sweet, J.A. (1989) 'Children's experiences in single-parent families: implications of cohabitation and marital transitions', *Family Planning Perspectives* 21(6): 256–60.

Burgess, A. (1997) *Fatherhood Reclaimed: The Making of the Modern Father*, London: Vermilion.

Burgess, A. (1998) *A Complete Parent: Towards a New Vision for Child Support*, London: IPPR.

Burgess, A. and Ruxton, S. (1996) *Men and Their Children: Proposals for Public Policy*, London: IPPR.

Burghes, L. (1991) *Supporting Our Children: The Family Impact of Child Maintenance*, London: Family Policy Studies Centre.

Burghes, L. (1993) *One-parent Families: Policy Options for the 1990s*, York: Joseph Rowntree Foundation.

Burghes, L. (1994) *Lone Parenthood and Family Disruption: The Outcomes for Children*, Occasional Paper 18, London: Family Policy Studies Centre.

Burghes, L., Clarke, L. and Cronin, N. (1997) *Fathers and Fatherhood in Britain*, Occasional Paper 23, London: Family Policy Studies Centre.

Burgoyne, C. and Millar, J. (1994) 'Enforcing child support obligations: the attitudes of separated fathers', *Policy and Politics* 22(2): 95–104.

Burgoyne, C.B. and Lewis, A. (1994) 'Distributive justice in marriage – equality or equity', *Journal of Community and Applied Social Psychology* 4(2): 101–14.

Burgoyne, J.L. and Clark, D. (1984) *Making a Go of It: A Study of Step Families in Sheffield*, London: Routledge and Kegan Paul.

Burns, A. (1995) 'Mother-headed families: here to stay', in J. Brannen and M. O'Brien (eds) *Parents and Children*, London: Institute of Education.

Burns, A. and Cairns, S. (1987) 'Mother headed families: A cross national comparison', *Australian Journal of Family Law* 1: 214–33.

Burrows, R. (1998) *The Dynamics of the Owner Occupied Market*, York: Centre for Housing Policy.

Cassetty, J. (1978) *Child Support and Public Policy*, Lexington, MA: Lexington Books.

Cheal, D. (1987) 'Showing them you love them: gift giving and the dialectic of intimacy', *Sociological Review*, 35: 150–69.

Cherlin, A. (1994) 'Stepfamilies: a reconsideration', Paper in International Convention on Changes in Family Patterns in Western Countries, Bologna, 6–8 October.

Cherlin, A.J., Furstenberg, F.F., Jr., Chase-Lansdale, P.L., Kiernan, K.E., Robins, P.K., Morrison, D.R. and Teller, J.O. (1991) 'Longitudinal studies of effects of divorce on children in Great Britain and the United States', *Science* 252: 1386–9.

Chief Child Support Officer (1994) *Annual Report*, Central Adjudication Services 93–94, London: HMSO.

Chief Child Support Officer (1995) *Annual Report*, Central Adjudication Services 94–95, London: HMSO.

Chief Child Support Officer (1996) *Annual Report*, Central Adjudication Services 95–96, London: HMSO.

Child Support (Miscellaneous Amendments Provisions) Regulations 1994 (SI 1994 No. 227).

Child Support Agency (July 1994) *The First Two Years*, Annual Report for 93/94 and Business Plan for 95/96, London: HMSO.

Child Support Agency (March 1995) *Business Plan 1995–96*, London: HMSO.

Child Support Agency (July 1995) *Annual Report 1994/1995*, London: HMSO. (Includes National Audit Office Report for 1994/95; Annual Accounts for 1994/95.)

Child Support Agency (1996) *Annual Report 1995/1996*, London: HMSO.

Child Support Agency (1998) *Clients, Funds and Accounts*, HCP 313 97–98 (23 February 1998). (Includes Report From the Comptroller and Auditor General on Client Fund Account for 96/97.)

Chilman, C.S., Nunnally, E.N. and Cox, F.M. (eds) *Variant Family Forms*, Newbury Park: Sage.

Clark, D. and Haldane, D. (1990) *Wedlocked? Intervention and Research in Marriage*, Cambridge: Polity Press in association with Basil Blackwell.

Clarke, K., Craig, G. and Glendinning, C. (1993) *Children Come First? The Child Support Act and Lone Parent Families*, London: Barnardo's, The Children's Society, NCH Action for Children, NSPCC and Save The Children.

Clarke, K., Craig, G. and Glendinning, C. (1996a) *Small Change: The Impact of the Child Support Act on Lone Mothers and Children*, London: Family Policy Studies Centre.

Clarke, K., Craig, G. and Glendinning, C. (1996b) *Children's Views on Child Support: Parents, Families and Responsibilities*, London: The Children's Society.

Clarke, K., Glendinning, C. and Craig, G. (1994a) 'Child support, parental responsibility and the law: an examination of the implications of recent British legislation', in J. Brannen and M. O'Brien (eds) *Childhood and Parenthood*, Proceedings of ISA Committee for Family Research Conference on Children and Families, Institute of Education, University of London.

Clarke, K., Glendinning, C. and Craig, G. (1994b) *Losing Support: Children and the Child Support Act*, London: The Children's Society.

Clarke, L. (1997) 'Who are fathers: a socio-demographic profile', in L. Burghes, L. Clarke and N. Cronin (eds) *Fathers and Fatherhood in Britain*, Occasional Paper 23, London: Family Policy Studies Centre.

Clarke, L., Condy, A. and Downing, A. (1998) *Fathers: A Socio-demographic Profile*, London: Family Policy Studies Centre.

Coleman, D. (1996) 'Male fertility trends in industrial countries: theories in search of some evidence', Paper presented to the Seminar on Fertility and the Male Life Cycle in the Era of Fertility Decline, Mexico, 1995.

Collier, R. (1993) *Waiting Til Father Gets Home: Family Values and the Reconstruction of Fatherhood in Family Law*, Newcastle Law School.

Coltraine, S. and Hickman, N. (1992) 'The rhetoric of rights and needs – moral discourse in the reform of child custody and child support laws', *Social Problems* 39(4): 400–20.

Committee of Public Accounts (November 1995) *First Report on the Child Support Agency*, Session 95–96 HC 31, London: HMSO.

Corden, A. (undated) *Child Support Agency Good Cause Review: Interviews with Field Staff*, York: Social Policy Research Unit, University of York.

Corneau, G. (1991) *Absent Fathers, Lost Sons: The Search for Masculine Identity*, Boston and London: Shambhala.

Council of Europe (1995) *The Status and Role of Fathers – Family Policy Aspects*, 24th Session of the Conference of European Ministers Responsible for Family Affairs, Helsinki.

Cowan, C.P. (1988) 'Working with men becoming fathers: the impact of a couple group intervention', in P. Bronstein and C.P. Cowan (eds) *Fatherhood Today: Men's Changing Roles in the Family*, Chichester: Wiley.

Cowan, P.A. and Hetherington, M. (eds) (1991) *Family Transitions*, New Jersey: Lawrence Erlbaum Associates.

Craig, G., Clarke, K. and Glendinning, C. (1995) 'Child support savings or service?', *Benefits*, April/May.

Daly, K. (1995) 'Reshaping fatherhood: finding the models', in W. Marsiglio (ed.) *Fatherhood: Contemporary Theory, Research and Social Policy*, London: Sage.

Danish Ministry of Social Affairs (1993) *Fathers in Families of Tomorrow*, Copenhagen: Ministry of Social Affairs.

Davidoff, L. and Hall, C. (1987) *Family Fortunes*, London: Routledge.

Davis, G., Cretney, S. and Collins, J. (1994) *Simple Quarrels: Negotiating Money and Property Disputes in Divorce*, Oxford: Clarendon Press.

de Singly, F. (1993) 'The social construction of a new paternal identity', in *Fathers in Families of Tomorrow*, Report from conference in Copenhagen.

De'Ath, E. (ed.) (1992) *Stepfamilies*, Croydon: National Stepfamily Association, Significant Publications.

Delboca, D. and Flinn, C.J. (1994) 'Expenditure decisions of divorced mothers and income distribution', *Journal of Human Resources* 29(3): 742–61.

Dench, G. (1994) *The Frog and the Prince and the Problem of Men*, London: Neanderthal Books.

Dennis, N. and Erdos, G. (1992) *Families without Fatherhood*, London: IEA Health and Welfare Unit.

Depner, C.E. and Bray, J.H. (eds) (1993) *Non Residential Parenting*, Newbury Park: Sage.

Deutschmann, C. (1996) 'Construction: on the actuality of Marx and Simmel', in *Thesis Eleven* No. 47: 1–21.

Devault, M.L. (1989) 'Doing housework: feeding and family life', in G. Gerstel and G. Engell (eds) *Families at Work*, Philadelphia: Temple University Press.

DSS (1993) HC 69, *The Operation of the Child Support Act*, Social Security Select Committee First Report, London: HMSO.

DSS (1996) *The Requirement to Co-operate: A Report on the Operation of the 'Good Cause' Provisions*, DSS.

DSS (1998) *Child Support Agency Quarterly Summary of Statistics*, London: HMSO.

Duncan, S. and Kirby, K. (1983) *Preventing Rent Arrears*, London: HMSO.

Dunleavy, P. and O'Leary, B. (1991) *Theories of The State*, London: Macmillan.

Dunleavy, P., Gamble, A. and Peele, G. (1990) *Developments in British Politics*, Basingstoke: Macmillan.

Edwards, S. and Halpern, A. (1992) 'Parental responsibility: an instrument of social policy' *Family Law*, 113–18.

Eekelaar, J. (1991) *Regulating Divorce*, Oxford: Clarendon Press.

Eekelaar, J. and Maclean, M. (1986) *Maintenance After Divorce*, Oxford: Clarendon Press.

Eekelaar, J., Clive, E. with Clarke, K. and Raikes, S. (1977) *Custody After Divorce*, Oxford: SSRC Centre for Socio-Legal Studies.

Elliott, B.J. and Richards, M.P.M. (1991) 'Children and divorce: educational performance and behaviour before and after parental separation', *International Journal of Law and the Family* 15(3): 258–76.

Ermisch, J. (1990) 'Analysis of the dynamics of lone parenthood: socio–economic influences on entry and exit rates', in E. Dusk (ed.) *Lone Parent Families: The Economic Challenge*, Paris: OECD.

Ermisch, J. and Wright, R. (1989) *Welfare Benefits and Lone Parents' Employment*, Discussion Paper No. 159, London: NIESR.

Families Need Fathers (1990) *The Nurture of Children: The Response to 'Children Come First'*, London: FNF.

Finch, J. (1989) *Family Obligations and Social Change*, London: Polity Press.

Finch, J. and Mason, J. (1990) 'Divorce, remarriage and family obligations', *Sociological Review* 38(2): 219–46.

Finch, J. and Mason, J. (1993) *Negotiating Family Responsibilities*, London and New York: Tavistock/Routledge.

Fine, M.A. and Fine, D.R. (1994) 'An examination and evaluation of recent changes in divorce laws in five western countries – the critical role of values', *Journal of Marriage and the Family* 56(2): 249–63.

Firth, R., Hubert, J. and Forge, A. (1970) *Families and their Relatives*, London: Routledge and Kegan Paul.

Ford, J. (1997) 'Mortgage arrears, mortgage possessions and homelessness', in R. Burrows, N. Pleace and D. Quilgars (eds) *Homelessness and Social Policy*, London: Routledge.

Ford, J. and Kempson, E. (1997) *Bridging the Gap? Safety Nets for Mortgagors*, York: York Publishing Services.

Ford, J., Kempson, E. and Wilson, M. (1995) *Mortgage Arrears and Possessions: Perspectives from Borrowers, Lenders and the Courts*, London: HMSO.

Ford, R. and Millar, J. (eds) (1998) *Private Lives and Public Responses*, London: PSI.

Ford, R., Marsh, A. and Finlayson, L. (1998) *What Happens to Lone Parents*, London: The Stationery Office.

Ford, R., Marsh, A. and McKay, S. (1995) *Changes in Lone Parenthood*, DSS Research Report No. 40, London: HMSO.

Fox, G.L. (1981) 'Daughters of divorce: the roles of fathers and father-figures in the lives of adolescent girls following divorce', unpublished, quoted Fox, G.L. (1985).

Fox, G.L. (1985) 'Non custodial fathers', in S.M.H. Hanson and F.W. Bozett (eds) *Dimensions of Fatherhood*, London: Sage.

French, S. (ed.) *Fatherhood*, London: Virago.

Friedman, H.J. (1980) 'The father's parenting experience in divorce', *American Journal of Orthopsychiatry* 137: 1177–82.

Funder, K., Harrison, M. and Weston, R. (1993) *Settling Down: Pathways of Parents After Divorce*, Melbourne: Australian Institute for Family Studies.

Furstenberg, F.F., Jr. (1987) 'The new extended family: the experience of parents and children after remarriage', in K. Pasley and M. Ihinger-Tallman (eds) *Remarriage and Step-Parenting: Current Research and Theory*, New York: The Guildford Press.

Furstenberg, F.F., Jr. (1988a) 'Good dads – bad dads: two faces of fatherhood', in A.J. Cherlin (ed.) *The Changing American Family and Public Policy*, Washington, DC: The Urban Institute Press.

Furstenberg, F.F., Jr. (1988b) 'Marital disruptions, child custody, and visitation', in A. Kahn and S.B. Kamerman (eds) *Child Support: From Debt Collection to Social Policy*, London: Sage.

Furstenberg, F.F., Jr. (1995) 'Fathering in the inner city: paternal participation and public policy', in W. Marsiglio (ed.) *Fatherhood, Contemporary Theory, Research and Social Policy*, London: Sage.

Furstenberg, F.F., Jr. and Nord, C.W. (1985) 'Parenting apart: patterns of child rearing after marital disruption', *Journal of Marriage and the Family* 47: 893–904.

Furstenberg, F.F., Jr., Nord, C.W., Peterson, J.L. and Zill, N. (1983) 'The life course of children of divorce: marital disruption and parental conflict', *American Sociological Review* 48: 656–68.

Garfinkel, I., McLanahan, S., Seltzer, J.A. and Meyer, D.R. (1997) 'The effects of child support policy on non-resident fathers', Paper for Princeton conference, 1995.

Garfinkel, I., McLanacan, S., Meyer, D.R. and Seltzer, J.A. (eds) (1998) *Fathers Under Fire: The Revolution in Child Support Enforcement*, New York: Russell Sage.

Garnham, A. and Knights, E. (1994) *Putting the Treasury First*, London: CPAG.

Gibson, C.S. (1991) 'The future for maintenance', *Civic Justice Quarterly* 330–46.

Gibson, C.S. (1994) *Dissolving Wedlock*, London and New York: Routledge.

Giddens, A. (1992) *The Transformation of Intimacy*, London: Polity Press.

Giveans, D. and Robinson, M.K. (1985) 'Fathers and the preschool child', in S.M.H. Hanson and F.W. Bozett (eds) *Dimensions of Fatherhood*, London: Sage.

Goldstein, J., Freud, A. and Solnit, A.J. (1973) *Beyond the Best Interests of the Child*, New York: Free Press.

Gorell Barnes, G., Thompson, P., Daniel, G. and Burchardt, N. (1998) *Growing Up In Stepfamilies*, Oxford: Clarendon Press.

Goto, S.G. (1996) 'To trust or not to trust: situational and dispositional determinants', *Social Behaviour and Personality* 24(2): 119–32.

Greif, G.L. (1992) 'Lone fathers in the United States: an overview and practical implications', *British Journal of Social Work* 22: 565–74.

Greve, J. and Currie, E. (1990) *Homelessness in Britain*, York: JRMT Findings 10.

Haddad, T. (ed.) (1993) *Men and Masculinities: A Critical Anthology*, Toronto: Canadian Scholars Press.

Hafner, J. (1993) *The End of Marriage: Why Monogamy Isn't Working*, London: Century.

Hansard, House of Commons (1991) *Child Support Bill*, Issue No. 1560, 3–7 June, col. 178–249.

Hansard, House of Lords (1991) *Child Support Bill*, Issue No. 1496: 25–28 February, col. 774–839.

Haskey, J. (1989a) 'One parent families and their children in Great Britain: numbers and characteristics', *Population Trends* 55: 27–33.

Haskey, J. (1989b) 'Trends in marriage and divorce, and cohort analysis of the proportion of marriages ending in divorce', *Population Trends* 54: 21–8.

Haskey, J. (1998) 'One parent families and their dependent children', *Population Trends* 91: 5–15.

Haskey, J. and Kiernan, K. (1989) 'Cohabitation in Great Britain – characteristics and estimated numbers in cohabiting relationships', *Population Trends* 58: 23–32.

Hennis, M. (1995) 'Pressure squeeze: the impact of pressure groups on child support policy, post-implementation', unpublished MA Thesis, University of York.

Herlth, A. (1997) *Conditions of 'Successful' Paternal Behavior. Stability and Complexity*, European Observatory Seminar, Lisbon.

Herzog, E. and Sudig, C.E. (1971) *Boys in Fatherless Families*, Washington, DC: Government Printing Office.

Hess, R.D. and Camara, K.A. (1979) 'Post divorce family relations as mediating factors in the consequences of divorce for children', *Journal of Social Issues*, 35(4): 79–96.

Hetherington, E.M. (1972) 'The effects of father absence on personality development in adolescent daughters', *Developmental Psychology* 7: 313–26.

Hetherington, E.M. (1987) 'Family relations six years after divorce', in K. Pasley and M. Ihinger-Tallman (eds) *Remarriage and Step Parenting: Current Research and Theory*, New York: The Guildford Press.

Hetherington, E.M., Cox, M. and Cox, R. (1985) 'Long term effects of divorce and remarriage on the adjustment of children', *Journal of Child Psychiatry* 56: 518–30.

Hewitt, P. (1993) *About Time: the Revolution in Work and Family Life*, London: IPPR/Rivers, Oram Press.

Hills, M.S. (1992) 'Role of economic resources and remarriage in financial assistance for children of divorce', *Journal of Family Issues* 13(2): 158–78.

Hoggett, B. (1993) *Parents and Children*, London: Sweet and Maxwell.

Holmans, A. (1989) 'Divorce and housing demand and need', in P. Symon (ed.) *Housing and Divorce*, Glasgow: Centre for Housing Research.

Holmans, A. (1990) 'Housing demand and need generated by divorce', in P. Symon (ed.) *Housing and Divorce*, Glasgow: Glasgow Centre for Housing Research.

Holmans, A. (1995) *Housing Demand and Need in England 1991–2011*, York: Joseph Rowntree Foundation.

House of Commons, HC 983 i–ii (1 December 1993) *The Operation of the Child Support Act*, Social Security Committee First Report Session 1992–93, London: HMSO.

House of Commons, HC 470 i (15 June 1994) *The Operation of the Child Support Act: Proposals For Change*, Social Security Committee Minutes of Evidence Session 1993–94, London: HMSO.

House of Commons, HC 470 ii (22 June 1994) *The Operation of the Child Support Act: Proposals For Change*, Social Security Committee Minutes of Evidence Session 1993–94, London: HMSO.

House of Commons, HC 470 (26 October 1994) *The Operation of the Child Support Act: Proposals For Change*, Social Security Committee Fifth Report Session 1993–94, London: HMSO.

House of Commons, HC 50 (24 January 1996) *The Performance and Operation of the Child Support Agency*, Social Security Committee Second Report Session 1995–1996, London: HMSO.

House of Commons, HC 440 (26 June 1996) *Child Support: Good Cause and the Benefit Penalty*, Social Security Committee Fourth Report Session 1995–1996, London: HMSO.

House of Commons, HC 282 (12 March 1997) *Child Support*, Social Security Committee Fifth Report Session 1996–1997, London: The Stationery Office.

House of Commons Papers (1994) Appropriation Accounts 1993–94; Volume 9: Classes XII and XIII – Health and Office of Population, Censuses and Surveys and Social Security, HCP 670 ix (1993–94).

House of Commons Official Report (July 1996) *Draft Child Support (Miscellaneous Amendments) Regulations 1996*, Sixth Standing Committee on Delegated Legislation 1996, London: HMSO.

Humphrey, R. (ed.) (1996) *Families Behind the Headlines*, Newcastle: University of Newcastle upon Tyne.

Hutton, S., Carlisle, J. and Corden, A. (1997) 'Depth follow-up to the CSA National Client Survey', Working Paper DSS 1501, Social Policy Research Unit, University of York.

Ihinger-Tallman, M., Pasley, K. and Buehler, C. (1995) 'Developing a middle range theory of father involvement post divorce', in W. Marsiglio (ed.) *Fatherhood: Contemporary Theory, Research and Social Policy*, London: Sage.

Jacobs, E. and Douglas, G. (1994) *Child Support: The Legislation*, Supplement to the third edition, London: Sweet and Maxwell.

Jacobson, D.S. (1978) 'The impact of marital separation/divorce on children: parent child separation and child adjustment', *Journal of Divorce* 1: 341–60.

Jensen, A.M. (1995) 'Paradoxes of fatherhood illustrated by the Norwegian case', in J. Brannen and M. O'Brien (eds) *Children and Parents*, Proceedings of ISA Committee for Family Research Conference on Children and Families 1994, London: Institute of Education.

Jones, H. and Millar, J. (eds) (1996) *The Politics of the Family*, Aldershot: Avebury.

Jordan, B., Redley, M. and James, S. (1994) *Putting the Family First*, London: UCL Press.

Jowell, A., Curtice, J., Brook, L. and Ahrendt, D. (1994) *British Social Attitudes 11th Report*, Dartmouth.

Kier, C. and Lewis, C. (1995) 'Family dissolution: mothers' accounts', in J. Brannen and M. O'Brien (eds) *Parents and Children*, Proceedings of ISA Committee for Family Research Conference on Children and Families 1994, London: Institute of Education.

Kiernan, K. (1990) *What about the Children?*, Family Policy Bulletin No. 3, London: Family Policy Studies Centre.

Kiernan, K. (1992) 'Men and women at work and home', *British Social Attitudes*.

Kiernan, K. and Wicks, M. (1990) *Family Change and Future Policy*, London: Family Policy Studies Centre.

Knijn, T. (1993) *Towards Post-Paternalism? Social and Theoretical Changes in Fatherhood*, WORC: Tilburg University.

Kruk, E. (1992) 'Psychological and structural factors contributing to the engagement of noncustodial fathers after divorce', *Family Conciliation Courts Review* 30: 81–101.

Kuhn, T.S. (1962) *The Structure of Scientific Revolutions*.

Kunz, J. (1992) 'The effects of divorce in children', in S.J. Bahr (ed.) *Family Research: A 60-Year Review 1939–1990*, New York: Lexicon Books.

Lamb, M.E. (1982) *Non-Traditional Families*, London: Lawrence Erlbaum.

Lamb, M.E. (1986) *The Father's Role: Applied Perspective*, New York: John Wiley.

Lamb, M.E. (ed.) (1997) *The Role of the Father in Child Development*, 3rd edn, New York: John Wiley.

Lambert, L. and Streather, J. (1980) *Children in Changing Families*, London: National Children's Bureau.

LaRossa, R. (1988) 'Fatherhood and social change', *Family Relations* 37: 451–8.

Lee, R.M. (1993) *Doing Research on Sensitive Topics*, London: Sage.

Leeming, A., Unell, J. and Walker, R. (1994) *Lone Mothers*, DSS Research Report No. 30, London: HMSO.

Leonard, D. and Hood-Williams, J. (1987) *Families*, Basingstoke and London: Macmillan.

Lewis, C. (1993) 'Mothers' and fathers' roles: similar or different', in *Fathers in Families of Tomorrow*, Conference proceedings, Copenhagen.

Lewis, C. and O'Brien, M. (1987) 'Constraints on fathers: research, theory and clinical practice', in C. Lewis and M. O'Brien (eds) *Reassessing fatherhood*, London: Sage.

Lister, R. (1994) 'The Child Support Act: shifting family financial obligations in the United Kingdom', *Social Politics: International Studies of Gender, State and Society* 1(2): 211–22.

Lister, R. (1995) 'Back to the family: family policies and politics under the Major Government', in H. Jones and J. Millar (eds) *The Politics of the Family*, Avebury: SPA.

Lloyd, T. (1996) 'Fathers in the media: an analysis of newspaper coverage of fathers and men as carers', in P. Moss (ed.) *Father Figures: Fathers in the Families of the 1990s*, Children In Scotland, Edinburgh: HMSO.

Lloyd, T. and Wood, T. (eds) (1987) *What Next For Men?*, London: Working With Men.

Lord Chancellor's Department (1995) *Looking to the Future: Mediation and the Ground for Divorce – The Government's Proposals*, London: HMSO.

Lowerson, R. (1997) 'Cutting both ways? The impact of Child Support Agency involvement on the work incentives of unemployed absent parents', MA dissertation, Department of Social Policy and Social Work, University of York.

Lund, M. (1987) 'The non-custodial father: common challenges in parenting after divorce', in C. Lewis and M. O'Brien (eds) *Reassessing Fatherhood*, New York: Sage.

Mac An Ghaill, M. (ed.) (1996) *Understanding Masculinities*, Buckingham: Open University Press.

McAdoo, J.L. (1986a) 'A black perspective on the father role in child development', *Marriage and Family Review* 9(3/4): 117–33.

McAdoo, J.L. (1986b) 'The role of black fathers', in H. McAdoo (ed.) *Black Families*, Los Angeles: Sage Publications.

McCarthy, P. (1994) 'Housing and post divorce parenting', Paper presented to the Social Policy Association Conference, 12 July 1994, University of Liverpool.

McCarthy, P. and Simpson, B. (1991) *Issues in Post Divorce Housing*, Aldershot: Avebury.

McCarthy, P. and Walker, J. (1996) *Evaluating the Longer Term Impact of Family Mediation*, Newcastle upon Tyne: Relate Centre for Family Studies.

McCluskey, U. (1990) 'Money in marriage', *Journal of Social Work Practice* 4: 16–29.

Maccoby, E., Depner, C. and Mnookin, R. (1990) 'Co-parenting in the second year after divorce', *Journal of Marriage and the Family* 52(1): 141–55.

McDonald, P. (ed.) (1986) *Settling Up: Property and Income Distribution on Divorce in Australia*, Melbourne, Australia: Institute of Family Studies.

McGurk, H. and Glachan, M. (1987) 'Children's conceptions of the continuity of parenthood following divorce', *JCPP* 28: 427–35.

McKay, S. and Marsh, A. (1994) *Lone Parents and Work: The Effects of Benefits and Maintenance*, DSS Social Security Report No. 25, London: HMSO.

McKee, L. (1987) 'Households during unemployment: the resourcefulness of the unemployed', in J. Brannen and G. Wilson (eds) *Give and Take in Families*, London: Allen and Unwin.

McKee, L. and O'Brien, M. (1983) 'Interviewing men: taking gender seriously', in E. Gamarnikow and J. Purvis (eds) *The Public and the Private*, London: Heinemann.

McKenzie (1998) *The National Newsletter from Families Needs Fathers*, issue 34, February.

Maclean, A.T. (1992) *The Future of the Family*, Edinburgh: Saint Andrew Press.

Maclean, M. (1987) 'Households after divorce', in J. Brannen and G. Wilson (eds) *Give and Take in Families*, London: Allen and Unwin.

Maclean, M. (1990) 'Lone parent families: family law and income transfers', in *Lone Parent Families: The Economic Challenge*, OECD Social Policy Studies No. 8, Paris.

Maclean, M. (1991) *Surviving Divorce: Women's Resources after Separation*, Basingstoke: Macmillan.

Maclean, M. (1993) 'Resource allocation between first and second families in the UK', Paper: Population and Family in the Low Countries, Centre for Socio-Legal Studies, Wolfson College, Oxford.

Maclean, M. (1994) 'The making of the Child Support Act of 1991: Policy making at the intersection of law and social policy', *Journal of Law and Society* 21(4): 505–19.

Maclean, M. and Eekalaar, J. (1993) 'Child support: the British solution', *International Journal of Law and the Family* 7: 205–29.

Maclean, M. and Eekalaar, J. (1997) *The Parental Obligation: A Study of Parenthood Across Households*, Oxford: Hart.

Maclean, M. and Wadsworth, M.E.J. (1988) 'The interests of the child after parental divorce. A long-term perspective', *International Journal of Law and the Family* 2: 155–66.

Manning, N. and Ungerson, C. (1990) *Social Policy Review 1989–1990*, Essex: Longman.

Marsh, A. (undated) *Absent Parenthood*, mimeo, London: Policy Studies Institute.

Marsh, A. (1993) *Absent Parenthood*, London: Policy Studies Institute.

Marsh, A. and McKay, S. (1993) *Families Work and Benefits*, London: Policy Studies Institute.

Marsh, A., Ford, H. and Finlayson, L. (1997) *Lone Parents, Work and Benefits: the First Effects of the Child Support Agency to 1994*, DSS Report 61, London: HMSO.

Marsiglio, W. (1995) 'Fatherhood scholarship: an overview', in W. Marsiglio (ed.) *Fatherhood: Contemporary Theory, Research and Social Policy*, London: Sage.

May, K.A. (1991) 'Interview techniques in qualitative research: concerns and challenges', in J.M. Morse (ed.) *Qualitative Nursing Research*, London: Sage.

Mead, M. (1967) 'Fatherhood', in S.A. Richardson and A.F. Guttmacher (eds) *Childbearing – Its Social and Psychological Aspects*, Baltimore: Williams and Wilkins.

Morgan, D. (1996) *Family Connections*, Cambridge: Polity Press.

Morgan, P. (1995) *Farewell to the Family?*, London: IEA.

Morris, L. (1990) *The Workings of the Household*, London: Polity Press.

Morris, L. and Lyon, S. (1994) *Gender Relations in Public and Private: Changing Research Perspectives*, London: Macmillan.

Moss, P. (1996a) *Father Figures: Fathers in the Families of the 1990s*, Children In Scotland, Edinburgh: HMSO.

Moss, P. (1996b) 'Fathers and work', in A. Burgess and S. Ruxton (eds) *Men and their Children: Proposals for Public Policy*, London: IPPR.

Moss, P. and Brannen, J. (1986) 'Fathers in employment', in C. Lewis and M. O'Brien (eds) *Reassessing Fatherhood: New Observations on Fathers and the Modern Family*, London: Sage.

Murray, C. (1990) *The Emerging British Underclass*, London: Institute of Economic Affairs.

Nash, J. (1965) 'The father in contemporary culture and current psychological literature', *Child Development* 36: 261–97.

National Association of Citizens Advice Bureaux (1994) *Child Support: One Year On*, London: NACAB.

National Audit Office (1995) 'Child Support Agency', Memorandum by the Comptroller and Auditor-General to the House of Commons Public Accounts Committee, NAO, London: HMSO.

National Council of One Parent Families (1994) *The Child Support Agency's First Year: The Lone Parent Case*, London: NCOPF.

Neale, B. and Smart, C. (1995) 'The New Parenthood?: Discussions from the ESRC Project, The Legal and Moral Ordering of Households in Transition', GAPU Sociology and Social Policy Research Working Paper 13.

Neale, B. and Smart, C. (1997) 'Experiments with parenthood', *Journal of the British Sociological Association* 31(2)(May): 201–19.

Newman, M. (1992) *Stepfamily Realities*, Sydney: Doubleday.

Nissel, M. (1987) 'Social change and the life course', in G. Cohen (ed.) *Social Change and the Life Course*, London: Tavistock, and Basingstoke: Macmillan.

O'Brien, M. (1992) 'Changing conceptions of fatherhood', in U. Bjornberg (ed.) *European Parents in the 1990s: Contractions and Comparisons*, New Brunswick and London: Transaction Publishers.

Oakley, A. (1979) *On Becoming a Mother*, Oxford: Martin Robertson.

Office of Population Census and Surveys (Summer 1995) *Population Trends*, OPCS.

Parliamentary Commissioner for Administration (January 1995) *Investigations of Complaints Against the Child Support Agency*, Third Report from the Session 1994–95, HC 135, London: HMSO.

Parliamentary Commissioner for Administration (March 1995) *The Child Support Agency*, Third Report from the Select Committee Session 1994–95, HC, London: HMSO.

Parliamentary Commissioner for Administration (March 1996) *Investigations of Complaints Against the Child Support Agency*, Third Report from the Session 1995–96, HC 20, London: HMSO.

Parsons, T. and Bales, R.F. (1955) *Family Socialization and Interaction Process*, Riverside: New York Free Press.

Pasley, K. and Ihinger-Tallman, M. (eds) (1987) *Remarriage and Step-Parenting: Current Research and Theory*, New York: The Guildford Press.

Perlman, D. and Duck, S. (eds) (1987) *Intimate Relationships*, Newbury Park: Sage.

Pill, C.J. (1990) 'Step families: redefining the family', *Family Relations* 39: 186–93.

Pleck, J.M. (1987) 'American fathers in historical perspective', in M.S. Kinmel (ed.) *Changing Men: New Directions in Research on Men and Masculinities*, Newbury Park, CA: Sage.

Popay, J., Hearn, J. and Edwards, J. (eds) (1998) *Men, Gender Divisions and Welfare*, London and New York: Routledge.

Pratt, E. (1991) *Living in Sin?*, Southsea: St Simon's Church.

Price, S.J. and McKenny, P.C. (1988) *Divorce*, Family Studies Text 9, London: Sage Publications.

Pringle, K. (1995) *Men, Masculinities and Social Welfare*, London: UCL Press.

Rebelsky, F. and Hanks, C. (1971) 'Fathers' verbal interaction with infants in the first three months', *Child Development* 42: 63–8.

Rendall, S.M., Clarke, L., Peters, H.E., Ranjit, N. and Verropoulou, G. (1997) *Incomplete Reporting of Male Fertility in the United States and Britain*, Working paper, mimeo.

Richards, M. and Dyson, M. (1982) *Separation, Divorce and the Development of Children: A Review*, London: Department of Health and Social Security.

Rodgers, B. and Pryor, J. (1998) *Divorce and Separation: The Outcomes for Children*, York: Joseph Rowntree Foundation.

Roll, J. (1994) *Child Support*, Research Paper 94/20, House of Commons Library.

Rotunda, E.A. (1985) 'American fatherhood: a historical perspective', *American Behavioural Science* 29(1): 7–25.

Rowe, R. (1993) *The Welfare State in Britain Since 1945*, London: Macmillan.

Rutter, M. (1985) 'Resilience in the face of adversity: protective factors and resistance to psychiatric disorder', *British Journal of Psychiatry* 147: 598–611.

Rutter, M. (1987) 'Psychosocial resilience and protective mechanisms', *American Journal of Orthopsychiatry* 57: 316–31.

Rutter, M. (1988) 'Functions and consequences of relationships: some psychopathological considerations', in R.A. Hinde and J. Stevenson-Hinde (eds) *Relationships with Families: Mutual Influences*, Oxford: Clarendon Press.

Rutter, M.L. (1981) *Maternal Deprivation Reassessed*, Harmondsworth: Penguin.

Schaeffer, N.C., Seltzer, J.A. and Klawitter, M. (1991) 'Estimating nonresponse and response bias', *Sociological Methods and Research* 20(1): 30–59.

Segal, L. (1990) *Slow Motion: Changing Masculinities, Changing Men*, London: Virago.

Seltzer, J. (1991) 'Relationships between fathers and children who live apart: the father's role after separation', *Journal of Marriage and the Family* 53 (February): 79–101.

Seltzer, J.A (1994) 'Consequences of marital dissolution for children', *Annual Review of Sociology* 20: 235–66.

Seltzer, J.A. and Bianchi, S.M. (1988) 'Children's contact with absent parents', *Journal of Marriage and the Family* 50: 663–77.

Seltzer, J.A. and Brandreth, Y. (1994) 'What fathers say about involvement with children after separation', *Journal of Family Issues* 15(1): 49–77.

Seltzer, J.A., Schaeffer, N.C. and Charng, H.W. (1989) 'Family ties after divorce. The relationship between visiting and paying child support', *Journal of Marriage and the Family* 51: 1013–31.

Silverman, D. (1993) *Interpreting Qualitative Data: Methods for Analysing Talk, Text and Interaction*, London: Sage.

Simpson, B., McCarthy, P. and Walker, J. (1995) *Being There: Fathers After Divorce*, Newcastle upon Tyne: Relate Centre for Family Studies.

Skinner, C. (1994) 'Negotiation and reciprocity: a framework for understanding the views of separated fathers on their parental responsibilities', unpublished.

Skinner, C. (1996) *The Parental Obligations of Fathers Living Apart*, Progress Report, October.

Skinner, C. (1998) 'The symbolic meanings attached to child maintenance monies', unpublished.

Skynner, R. and Cleese, J. (1983) *Families and How to Survive Them*, London: Methuen.

Smart, C. (1989) *Feminism and the Power Of Law*, London: Routledge.

Smart, C. (1997) 'Wishful thinking and harmful tinkering? Sociological reflections on family policy', *Journal of Social Policy* 26(3): 301–21.

Smith, D. (1990) *Stepmothering*, Hemel Hempstead: Harvester Wheatsheaf.

Song, M. and Edwards, R. (1995) '"Babymothers": raising questions about perspectives on black lone motherhood', Paper presented at the Social Policy Association Annual Conference, 18–20 July 1995, Sheffield Hallam University.

Sorenson, E.J. (1997) 'A national profile of nonresident fathers and their ability to pay child support', *Journal of Marriage and the Family* 59(4): 785–97.

Southwell, M. (1985) 'Children, divorce and the disposal of the matrimonial home', *Family Law* 15.

Speak, S., Cameron, S. and Gilroy, R. (1997) *Young Single Fathers' Participation in Fatherhood: Bridges and Barriers*, London: Family Policies Studies Centre.

Speed, M. and Kent, N. (1996) *Child Support Agency National Client Satisfaction Survey 1995*, DSS Research Report No. 51, London: HMSO.

Speed, M. and Seddon, J. (1995) *Child Support Agency National Client Satisfaction Survey 1994*, London: HMSO.

Speed, M., Crane, J. and Rudat, K. (1994) *Child Support Agency National Client Satisfaction Survey 1993*, London: HMSO.

Speed, M., Roberts, C. and Rudat, K. (1993) *Child Support Unit National Client Satisfaction Survey 1992*, London: HMSO.

Spock, B. (1974) *A Fathers' Companionship*, Redbook 24.

Stepfamily (1990) *Children Come First: A Response to the Government White Paper on Child Support and The Child Support Agency*, London: National Stepfamily Association.

Stephens, L. (1996) 'Will Johnny see Daddy this week? An empirical test of three theoretical perspectives of post divorce contact', *Journal of Family Issues*, 17(4): 466–94.

Stone, L. (1990) *Road to Divorce*, Oxford: Oxford University Press.

Stryker, S. (1980) *Symbolic Interactionism: A Social Structural Version*, Menlo Park, CA: Benjamin/Cummins.

Sullivan, D. (1986) 'Housing movements of the divorced and separated', *Housing Studies*, 1: 35–47.

Sutton, T. (1996) 'A socio-economic approach to child support compliance', Paper presented at the Australian National Family Conference, Brisbane 1996.

Sweet, J.A. and Bumpass, L.L. (1987) *American Families and Households*, New York: Russell Sage.

Sweet, J.A., Bumpass, L.L. and Call, V. (1988) *The Design and Content of the National Survey of Families and Households*, NSFH Working Paper 12, Madison: University of Wisconsin, Centre for Demography and Ecology.

Symon, P. (1990) 'Marital breakdown, gender and home ownership: the owner occupied home in separation and divorce', in P. Symon (ed.) (1991) *Housing and Divorce*, Studies in Housing No. 4, Glasgow: Centre for Housing Research, University of Glasgow.

Thompson, E.H., Jr. (ed.) (1994) *Older Men's Lives*, London: Sage.

Thompson, L. and Walker, A.J. (1989) 'Gender in families: women and men in marriage, work and parenthood', *Journal of Marriage and the Family* 51: 845–71.

Thompson, P. (1995) 'Transmissions between generations', in J. Brannen and M. O'Brien (eds) *Parents and Children*, London: Institute of Education.

Tyrell, H. and Schulze, H.-J. (1997) *Stability as a Cultural Ingredient of Parenting*, Lisbon: European Observatory paper.

UK, Cmnd 1264 (1990) *Children Come First: The Government's Proposals on the Maintenance of Children*, London: HMSO.

UK, Cmnd 2469 (February 1994) *Child Support: Reply by the Government to the First Report on the Operation of the Child Support Act*, London: HMSO.

UK, Cmnd 2813 (1995) DSS, *The Government's Expenditure Plans 1995/96–1997/98*, London: HMSO.

UK, Cmnd 2865 (May 1995) *Reply by the Government to the Third Report from the Parliamentary Commissioner for Administration – Session 1994–95*, London: HMSO.

UK, Cmnd 3992 (July 1998) *Children First: A New Approach to Child Support*, London: The Stationery Office.

Vogler, C. and Pahl, J. (1994) 'Money, power and inequality within marriage', *Sociological Review* 42(2): 263–88.

Walker, J. (1992) 'Divorce, remarriage and parental responsibility', in E. De'Ath (ed.) *Step Families: What Do We Know? What Do We Need to Know?*, London: The National Stepfamily Association, Significant Publications.

Walker, J. (1996) *Staying in Touch*, Family Policy Studies Centre Bulletin, November.

Walker, J. and Hornick, J.P. (1996) *Communication in Marriage and Divorce*, London: BT Forum.

Walker, J., McCarthy, P. and Timms, N. (1994) *Mediation: The Making and Remaking of Co-operative Relationships*, Newcastle upon Tyne: Relate Centre for Family Studies.

Wallbank, J. (1997) 'The campaign for change of the Child Support Act 1991: reconstituting the "absent" father', *Social & Legal Studies* 6(2): 191–216.

Wallerstein, J.S. and Blakeslee, S. (1989) *Second Chances: Men, Women and Children a Decade after Divorce*, New York: Ticknor & Fields.

Wallerstein, J.S. and Kelly, J.B. (1980) *Surviving the Breakup: How Children and Parents Cope with Divorce*, New York: Basic Books.

Wedge, P. and Prosser, H. (1973a) *Born to Fail?*, London: Arrow Books in association with the National Children's Bureau.

Wedge, P. and Prosser, H. (1973b) *Children in Adversity*, London: Pan Books.

Weekly Hansard, House of Commons (1995) *Child Support Bill*, 20 March 1995, col. 21–110.

Weston, R. (1992) 'Income circumstances of parents and children: a longitudinal view', in K. Funder, M. Harrison and R. Weston (eds) *Settling Down: Pathways of Parents After Divorce*, Melbourne: Australian Institute of Family Studies.

Wheelock, J. (1990) *Husbands at Home*, London: Routledge.

White Franklin, A. (ed.) (1983) *Family Matters*, Oxford: Pergamon Press.

Whitehead, B.D. (1993) 'Dan Quayle was right', *Atlantic Monthly* April.

Wilson, G. (1987) 'Money: patterns of responsibility and irresponsibility in marriage', in J. Brannen and G. Wilson (eds) *Give and Take in Families*, London: Allen and Unwin.

Wofram, S. (1987) *In-laws and Out-laws: Kinship and Marriage in England*, London: Croom Helm.

Wolcott, I. and Glezer, H. (1995) *Work and Family Life*, Melbourne: Australian Institute of Family Studies.

Young, M. and Wilmot, P. (1973) *The Symmetrical Family*, London: Routledge and Kegan Paul.

Zelizer, A. (1994) *The Social Meaning of Money*, New York: Basic Books.

Zelizer, A. (1996) 'Payments and social ties', *Sociological Forum* 11(3): 481–95.

Index

Note: past partners from child-bearing relationships of any status are included in the index under 'mothers'.
CSA in index entries refers to Child Support Agency